# THE COMPLETE
# RELAXATION
## BOOK

# THE COMPLETE
# RELAXATION
# BOOK

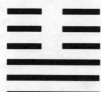

## A Manual of Eastern and Western Techniques

## JAMES HEWITT

RIDER
LONDON

First published in 1982 as *Relaxation East & West* by Rider

An imprint of Random Century Group Limited
20 Vauxhall Bridge Road, London SW1V 2SA

Reissued as *The Complete Relaxation Book* in 1986
Reprinted 1989, 1990, 1991, 1992

Random Century Australia (Pty) Limited
20 Alfred Street, Milsons Point,
Sydney, NSW 2061, Australia

Random Century New Zealand Limited
18 Poland Road, Glenfield,
Auckland 10, New Zealand

Random Century South Africa (Pty) Limited
PO Box 337, Bergvlei, South Africa

Printed and bound in Great Britain by
The Guernsey Press Co. Ltd, Guernsey, Channel Islands.

A catalogue record for this book is available from the British Library.

ISBN  0-7126-3096-1

This book is printed on recycled paper.

# Contents

# *Preface*

Looking now at the contents of my youthful works on relaxation and at the plan of the present volume, I discern two main differences. Missing in the earlier works were the presentation of meditation as a method of deep relaxation, and, apart from tentative pointers, discussion of what might be called relaxation's wider dimensions. These were discoveries I made later, through study and practice.

The 'relaxation' that is the subject of this book is not relaxation in the popular usage of the word, as a transient respite from work and from the cares and responsibilities of living. This book is about deep psychophysical relaxation – which scientific investigation shows to be deeper in several ways than deep sleep – and about carrying relaxation into everyday thought, feeling and activity, manifested as poised living.

It is connected, too, with the profoundest experiences known to human consciousness, however you choose to interpret them. Relaxation followed right through offers a way – even a 'Way' in the Eastern sense of a mystical 'path' – to expansion of consciousness, to greater freedom from conditioning, to spiritual unfoldment and experiential wisdom.

## THE BOOK IN OUTLINE

Chapter 1 states the aims of this book: to describe practical methods from both East and West to induce deep states of relaxation and to show how relaxation can be the basis for an art of poised living, which can be achieved despite the stressful nature of modern life. Poised living is not just a health-protection method or a therapy. It is a lifestyle for the development of full humanness (self-actualization) and for letting go and opening up to mindfulness of being.

Chapter 2 describes progressive relaxation, the primary Western therapeutic method of deep muscular relaxation. Relaxation is taught here as a neuromuscular skill, which can be learned like any other, such as buttoning a coat or driving a car. By developing your kinaesthetic sense, or muscle awareness, you can learn to recognize tension in the skeletal muscles and to let go from it – that is, relax the muscles. This is done progressively from toes to scalp; the muscles controlling speech and imagery, associated with thinking, may also be relaxed.

Chapter 3 is concerned with the application of muscular relaxation skill in everyday activities, using minimum effort for maximum effect. Muscles not essential for any action should be relaxed (differential relaxation). Energy is saved, efficiency increased.

Chapter 4 gives instruction in self-hypnosis, with suggestions for deep relaxation. It should be noted that all hypnosis is in a sense auto-hypnosis, as the cooperation of the subject is essential. Self-hypnosis can be learned by most people and the mind's remarkable capacity to respond to implanted suggestions harnessed for dissolving tensions, changing habits, treating illnesses, inducing confidence, self-improvement and for personal growth.

Chapter 5 discusses autogenic training which has attracted much interest in Europe, although therapists in Britain and the USA have been slower to use it. It resembles both progressive relaxation and self-hypnosis and uses auto-suggestion to induce feelings of muscle heaviness, warmth and so on.

Chapter 6 describes the instrumental techniques used to monitor our biological function. Biofeedback belongs to our technological age. It is a kind of push-button self-mastery, giving Yogin-like powers over body functions normally beyond voluntary control. Although the subject is not sure how he or she is doing it, brainwave rhythms can be altered, blood pressure lowered, and deep relaxation induced – all in response to monitored signals on electrical instruments. A principle of 'let it happen' is the key to success, just as it is in all relaxation methods and in Eastern tranquillity practices.

Chapter 7 describes the important techniques of poised posture and poised breathing. If the body is carried well and harmoniously balanced, actions are performed with the minimum of fatigue, and the lungs and other internal organs have room to function well. Body posture also influences inner posture. In this chapter we see how Zen posture and the Alexander method may be combined.

Chapter 8 describes methods of meditation that are acceptable to everyone: simple techniques that calm body and mind. The physiology of meditation has been studied by Western scientists who have found it to be one of the simplest ways of eliciting the 'relaxation response'. Some people see meditation as a way to higher consciousness or to enlightenment.

Chapter 9 deals with the continuing benefits of meditation in day-to-day living. Any activity in daily life can become a medium for meditation awareness. Mindfulness or bare attention is a mental hygiene, defeating stress, heightening perception and triggering peak experiences, which develops detachment and self-knowledge.

Chapter 10 opens with an account of how auto-suggestion may be used in states of deep relaxation which give contact with the unconscious mind. Relaxation is an essential preliminary to the manifestation of most so-called paranormal powers. When the conscious mind and will are pacified, the deep-seated true will may emerge. Relaxation is also the essence of the peak experience – moments of delight, meaning, and ego-transcendence. Mystical experience may be viewed as the ultimate relaxation experience. The chapter concludes with a discussion of altered consciousness and the possibility of higher states of consciousness.

Chapter 11 outlines the strategy for the use of the relaxation practices and gives a picture of the likely attitudes, psychology, philosophy and world view of the man or woman realizing a poised life. The characteristics of poised living are largely those described by Abraham H. Maslow for self-actualizing people. Peace of mind can be sustained in 'plateau living'. Poised living finds inspiration in philosophical Taoism, which teaches a special feeling for Nature and letting go to life's flow. The spirit of philosophical Taoism continues to animate Zen. Ordinary living is effortless flow and constant celebration.

# 1 Letting Go for Life

This book is a manual of instruction in the art of relaxation, or *letting go*, at various levels, employing techniques from both Western therapies and Eastern mystical traditions in a fruitful synthesis.

The practice of letting go releases tension from body and mind and opens up awareness – thereby improving health and protecting against disease, conserving and integrating energy, enhancing psychophysical skills, and promoting psychophysical poise. Letting go is essential to tapping the deep-rooted powers of the unconscious mind and to expansion of the mind's reaches. At its highest cultivation, letting go from the tension-knot that is the ego or I-process triggers the freedom, spontaneity and enlightenment that is the ultimate goal of the mystical traditional systems.

## THE ESOTERIC PSYCHOLOGIES

It should be noted that the mystical religions of the East are primarily esoteric psychologies, using meditation supported by postural training and the cultivation of certain ego-dropping attitudes, to attain enlightenment and a transformation of the quality of consciousness. The paths they describe are open to all, and in the last twenty years or so Western interest in them has grown considerably.

Letting go is at the heart of practice in these traditions and has a major influence on the generation of poised attitudes.

Physical poise is promoted in the East by smooth, flowing body exercises and by postural training, such as are found in Indian Hatha Yoga and the Chinese slow-motion movements Tai chi ch'uan. Yoga body exercises – really postures that are held motionless – have become popular with many Western men and women, who, when asked the practical benefits derived from such practice, always mention the relaxation they induce. Body and mind are brought into harmony through such exercises, but the effectiveness of Eastern body–mind training becomes immeasurably greater when the body controls and postural realignments are practised together with meditation and the cultivation of poised attitudes to Nature, to other people, and to living. Then the full dimensions of these Eastern systems are revealed and may be incorporated in poised living.

In this book I have drawn eclectically on techniques and attitudes from the Eastern psychologies – in particular from Hindu Vedanta, Buddhism, Taoism and Zen. Taoism and Zen are especially valuable in supplying methods and attitudes conducive to poised living and integrated wellbeing. Philosophical Taoism, most of all, provides inspiration and shapes our overall attitudes and practices, while Zen, which philosophical Taoism influenced, provides practical techniques for poise of body and mind. Zen is itself a practical way of life, and views body and mind as a unity.

## FOLLOWING THE TAO

In this book I am attempting to establish what could be viewed as a practical basis for a kind of Western Taoism. By Taoism I mean what is generally called 'philosophical Taoism' and not the religion of that name. Philosophical Taoism has only four important 'scriptures'. They are the works of Lao Tzu, Chuang Tzu, Lieh Tzu and Huai-nan Tsu. Lao Tzu's aphoristic *Tao Te Ching* is an inspiration for any person who values poised living, and the *Book of Chuang Tsu* is a witty and wise commentary upon Lao Tsu's work, as well as being a classic exposition of philosophical Taoism in its own right.

All things belong to the One, to the all-pervasive Tao. Tao is the silent, ineffable power and intelligence of the universe, supplying its life-energy and its forms, though it is itself formless.

'To adjust oneself to events and surroundings casually [i.e. with naturalness and relaxation] is the Way of Tao,' Chuang Tsu stated. Philosophical Taoists taught that one should live calmly, cheerfully and compassionately; that true strength lay in gentleness and true will in letting go and not-forcing. The wise life style is to work and live in harmony with Nature's laws. Their views on protecting the balance of nature are echoed today by the ecologists, and their views on the nature of the universe have affinities with the findings of modern physics. Joy is found in natural spontaneity and in being fully human. Be passive like a mirror and respond to surroundings like an echo to a sound. Calm acceptance leads to a sense of unity with what is. One seeks to live as naturally as rain falls, grass grows and fish swim.

He who follows Tao is strong of body, clear of mind and sharp of sight and hearing. He does not clutter up his mind with worries, and is flexible in his adjustment to external conditions. The heaven cannot help being high, the earth cannot help being wide . . . and all things of the creation cannot help but live and grow. (Chuang Tsu)

Following the Tao is one way of describing the way of poise and relaxation.

## ZEN

The philosophy and practice of Taoism found a congenial home in the empirical Ch'an (Japanese, Zen) Buddhism. The Zen masters teach letting go as the basis of seeing into one's nature, and of finding unity with Nature and the Universe. The supreme Zen enlightenment experience of 'satori' (or kensho) is the ultimate letting go, the ultimate relaxation experience, charged by the realization of one's essential unity with the One, the Tao. Robert Linssen, in *Living Zen* (p. 288), writes: 'No satori is possible without relaxation of body, emotion, and thought.'

A common enlightenment experience is reported by people of different races and cultural traditions. Interpretations vary: theist, non-theist, pantheist, mystical, non-mystical, religious, non-religious, and so on. But whatever the interpretation – what William James called 'overbelief' – there remains the *experience*. There is a common psychological experience and great similarities of technique for eliciting it. The essence of the experience is a profound relaxation: the stripping away or jettisoning of illusions and inessential burdens.

Sages throughout the centuries have spoken or written of the need to let go from or drop the ego or I-process, with all its attachments, cravings, defences and clung-to possessions. You have to relax ego-striving and ego-tension and make yourself open and available for the liberating experience, which is experiential knowledge of what Thomas Merton called 'the ground of openness': that which Eastern esoteric psychologists call an 'emptiness' and which is paradoxically a fullness. Alan Watts wrote, in *Beyond Theology*, that ultimate faith 'is not in or upon anything at all. It is complete letting go.' Krishnamurti put it: 'You cannot choose Reality. Reality must choose you.' This requires relaxation and open awareness. Poised attention without self-projecting leads to awareness of the workings of the I-process and to the possibility of an abrupt and total unmasking, so that you see, as the Zenists say, your original face or true (Buddha) nature.

Intellectual people tend to look to Jnana Yoga, the path of self-inquiry, for methods to reach enlightenment. Here the key question is: 'Who or what am I?' Devotional temperaments favour Bhakti Yoga, the path of surrender to something infinitely greater than oneself. These two approaches are found in all the major mystical traditions; both require letting go, for the former approach sees through the phoniness and pettiness of the ego, so that it is let go from or dropped.

# MEDITATIVE AWARENESS

Bare awareness is the solvent that removes the ego's tensions and its defensive armour. According to the Eastern traditional psychologies, behind the 'I' that has been built up by thought, memory, feelings, and social conditioning lies pure consciousness, the ground of being. It is the task of meditation to reveal it.

There are two kinds of meditation practice. The first kind occurs in motionless sitting, usually in a posture conducive to effortless and poised use of the meditation method. The other kind of meditation accompanies everyday activities, which become infused with the clarity and peacefulness of pure awareness and being.

Thought is not suppressed during meditation, but psychological devices, in which passive awareness is the main component, are used which quieten the mind. The methods described in chapter 8 for sitting meditation can be used by any reader and will prove beneficial in deeply relaxing body and mind and in cultivating clarity of consciousness. The succeeding chapter shows how mindfulness or bare attention can achieve similar results in daily activities. The pure quality of consciousness during the sitting periods will also infuse ordinary activities, whatever they may be, particularly in the period immediately following meditation.

One result of learning bare attention is that perception becomes direct, with a minimum of interference and distortion from thoughts and accompanying feelings. For most people, awareness of grass and tree and cloud, of sunlight and air on skin, and of feelings, are through the words by which they name these things. Their perception is not direct, but conceptual.

Direct perception is a keynote of Zen experience, by which perception of the 'ordinary' is enhanced and becomes 'marvellous'. There is a heightened sense of reality when awareness centres lucidly in the present.

## FREE, SPONTANEOUS AND OPEN

Dr D. T. Suzuki, the greatest expert on Zen to write in English, said that the aim of Zen training is to set us free from all forms of bondage. This is true of all the esoteric psychologies and we have seen that these psychologists regard the ego, with its projections, cravings and defences, as the major cause of illusion and captivity. A sense of freedom also comes through using the body with natural efficiency, eliminating unnecessary tensions so that perceptions, feelings and the mental life can flow effortlessly.

As a symbol for Nature, the Chinese use a phrase, *tzu-jan*, meaning 'of itself so'. So each individual consciousness, being *of* nature and *of* the universe, as well as *in* them, is itself so. Hence the importance of naturalness and spontaneity in Taoism and Zen, and in the arts and sports influenced by them.

It is important not to strive for results, which is the ego's principal activity. Then consciousness is found to be effortless, of itself so, and silence, stillness and space or emptiness the true nature of the mind. Then feelings and sensations come and go like wild geese crossing an expanse of clear sky; open awareness reflects them but does not struggle either to deflect them or to try to retain them. So also with thoughts. This is a new mode of consciousness for most people, but one whose profound value will be appreciated once it has been experienced even momentarily.

There is a danger that is easily overlooked; in recognizing the importance of letting go and of no longer forcing the mind to behave in certain ways or to stop behaving in certain ways, we make the mistake of making an effort not to be effortful. Success in letting go from tension in the body muscles will show the way to avoid this trap, for the same problem exists in attaining relaxation at any level, and practice in muscular relaxation makes a sound basis for learning the art of letting go, which is what relaxation is.

Awareness in poised living is open primarily to the living moment, to the continuous process of birth in the present, which means opening up to a greatly increased sense of reality.

Thus the cultivation of increased openness, relaxation and psychophysical poise is not just a way of releasing stress and improving health, but a way of self-actualizing, of expanding consciousness and of experiencing reality more directly and intensely.

Once relaxation and spontaneity in living have been tasted, all manner of paradoxes make living sense: that by losing one's self one finds one's Self; that the profound seriousness of living is best recognized by living lightly (without unnecessary physical or psychological burdens); that we can play the game of fighting the things we dislike, while recognizing at the same time the necessity for their presence as part of the total scheme of things, of the interplay of the opposites, the *yin* and the *yang* of the Chinese universal view. That the best 'means' of achieving supreme wellbeing is by 'no means', by simply letting go.

With right relaxation and open awareness, morality takes care of itself, unforced. Compassion and other valuable and harmonious qualities arise as a natural outcome of poised, spontaneous living. The free, relaxed person experiences wellbeing in doing what is right.

The discovery of natural moral wisdom is matched by the discovery of natural body wisdom. The practice of relaxation helps the body discover its natural instinctive wisdom, which in turn favours body–mind harmony and unity. That is why a Japanese person interested in Zen will often train in judo, swordsmanship or archery, or some other Zen-influenced physical art.

The characteristics of people experienced in the art of poised living, as I see the art, are largely similar to those Abraham H. Maslow described for what he called 'self-actualizing' people; people who actualize natural human growth potential. Prominent among these characteristics are openness, naturalness, spontaneity, autonomy, acceptance, creativity, capacity to love, a strong sense of reality, and ego-transcendence. Not for nothing did Professor Maslow frequently use the word 'Taoist' to describe the process of self-actualization and the personality of self-actualizers.

The self-actualizing person, according to Maslow, is likely to

be familiar with 'peak experiences': moments of intense transcendental delight. When very intense, such experiences are
sometimes described as 'mystical', or as examples of people
experiencing 'higher consciousness'. I state with some confidence that mastery of the art of poised living generates
Taoist/self-actualizing characteristics and triggers more peak
experiences, or the capacity to spend long periods at a higher
'plateau' level. A discussion of these matters will be found in
chapter 11.

Poised living is accessible to everyone, regardless of belief,
with the exception of fanaticism or ideological rigidities.
Acceptance, tolerance, what Wordsworth called 'a wise passivity', and openness to being are integral parts of a poised
approach to living. When you are oriented toward 'being'
rather than 'having', things are done and enjoyed for their own
sakes rather than for what the ego can get out of them.

## LIVING POETICALLY

Maslow's 'self-actualization' is not the only term for living
used by a philosopher and psychologist that relates to my concept of *poised living*.

There is Dr Erich Fromm's use of 'well-being', defined by
him on p. 91 of *Zen Buddhism and Psychoanalysis* (Harper and
Row):

Well-being is the state of having arrived at the full development of
reason: reason not in the sense of a merely intellectual judgment, but
in that of grasping truth by 'letting things be' (to use Heidegger's
term) as they are. Well-being is possible only to the degree to which
one has overcome one's narcissism; to the degree to which one is
open, responsive, sensitive, awake, empty (in the Zen sense). Well-
being means to be fully related to man and nature affectively, to
overcome separateness and alienation, to arrive at the experience of
oneness with all that exists . . . it means also to be creative. . . .'

In Dr D. T. Suzuki's contribution to the same book, he uses
the expression 'artist of life'. The artist of life lives creatively in

the here-and-now, every moment a birth, free as the wind, having let go from a self encased in egocentric existence. Dr Suzuki said that the true artist of life was described succinctly by the Zen master T'ang: 'With a man who is master of himself wherever he may be found he behaves truly to himself' (pp. 15–16).

There is also R. H. Blyth's use of the word 'poetical'. 'The way of poetry,' wrote Professor Blyth, in *Zen and Zen Classics* (Hokuseido Press, vol. 1, p. 17), '. . . consists in giving the highest possible value to every moment.' And (p. 21): 'What we have to do is not live traditionally or nationalistically or Asiatically or Christianically or Buddhistically or Zennically, but poetically – whatever that may mean in actual practice.'

All the terms discussed refer to living with relaxation and poise. Maslow was very aware that the attitudes he attributed to 'self-actualizing' people were 'Taoist'. Fromm in his last years found that humanistic psychology had much to learn from Zen, and when Suzuki spoke about 'artists of life' he had living by Zen in mind. Blyth wrote of 'living poetically' in a Zen context.

The message of Taoism and Zen is that the human organism can be trusted to regulate itself spontaneously and efficiently in a state of open awareness, sensitive, awake and alert, and relaxed to the immediate moment without trying either to repel or to wrest anything out of it. This is the state of mind which the Chinese call *wu-wei*, meaning 'not-interfering' or 'not-forcing'.

The greatest value of poised living is that even so-called 'ordinary' living is transformed. Zen master Ummon, in the tenth century, preached a sermon – 'Every day is a fine day.' Thoreau, at Walden in the nineteenth century, put it slightly differently when he wrote of 'a perpetual morning . . . morning is when I am awake and there is a dawn in me.' Thoreau was being an artist of life when he stated, 'Living is so dear, I did not wish to live what was not life,' and 'To affect the quality of the day, that is the highest of arts.'

Wellbeing is choosing life rather than continuing with a dead automatism, and it is made possible through letting go and opening up, through relaxation and psychophysical poise. It is allowing and creating the right conditions for growth to full humanness. Growth includes the unfoldment of those powers and the expansion of consciousness described in chapter 10.

## RELAXATION METHODS

Letting go at a psychical level is greatly facilitated and given a solid base for practice by acquiring skill in muscular relaxation. Various Western techniques for inducing deep muscular and mental relaxation are described in the first half of this book. You can experiment and discover those which work best for you.

By practising one or more of these body–mind relaxation methods, the effects on your mental life are soon experienced, and you become aware of the profound significance of altering the quality of consciousness. A new note is heard: it is the call to freedom from anxiety and conditioning that brings emancipation from egocentric existence. In the esoteric psychologies, this freedom is called enlightenment.

> Empty, lucid, self-illumined,
> With no over-exertion of the power of the mind.
>                         (Sengtsan, The *Hsinhsinming*)

Western and Eastern methods of psychophysical relaxation work well together. The benefits from such a practical synthesis are available to all, and are possible even in the teeth of the stress disease epidemic now gripping Western civilization.

## STRUGGLING WITH STRESS

Modern man is battling to establish a healthful state of equilibrium between himself and his environment. His psychophysical organism is called upon to adapt to rapid changes and to numerous severe and unprecedented stressors, which are

both physical and psychological, both obvious and hid
Though making life easier for people in some respects, the ra
development of technology in the twentieth century has
brought its own peculiar stresses of complexity, competition
and change. Ordinary life today is dangerously stressful for
millions of the citizens of the world's most developed nations.

The signs of inability to relax are ubiquitous in modern
society. As industrialization and technology spreads – dehu-
manizing, depersonalizing, and pressurizing – the symptoms of
so-called 'nervous tension' become more apparent. Some of the
obvious symptoms are anxiety, nervous troubles, headaches,
muscular aches and pains, insomnia, jitteriness, restlessness,
dependence on drugs, alcohol and tobacco, and the inability to
'unwind' even when the conditions are favourable. There are,
too, numerous psychosomatic disorders and diseases, often
unrecognized for what they are.

Doctors report that more than half the patients seen in
general practice often display puzzling symptoms that may be
attributed to the effects of stress. The incidence of 'mystery illnesses' is growing. Stress undermines the body's defences and
disease strikes at the weakest points. Hypertension or high
blood pressure is probably the most serious effect of tension,
because its symptoms may stay hidden for years. It leads to
narrowed arteries and to heart disease, so that suddenly and
without warning the hypertensive person may be struck down
by a heart attack or a stroke. One hundred years ago heart
attacks were rare in any age group: now young as well as old are
common victims.

Stress is 'the modern disease', or dis-ease. Distinguished
physicians in America and in Europe warn that stress is a major
killer.

## THE ANTIDOTE FOR STRESS

Drugs are not the answer to stress. At best, they are palliatives;
they do not get to the root of the problem. One becomes depen-
dent on them, and there are often harmful side-effects.

*Relaxation – deep muscular relaxation and the cultivation of poise in every department of living – is the natural way of releasing tension and the effective antidote against stress.*

The 'fight-or-flight response' has been described in many books and in newspaper and magazine articles. We perceive a threat to body or ego – our body mobilizes all its forces for fighting the threat or for running away from it. Mobilization means increases – in heart rate, blood pressure, metabolism (burning fuel), and so on. The trouble is that while actual fight or flight makes use of the body mobilization, the nature of modern life for most people gives few outlets for real fight or flight and the threats are daily and numerous. The body stays keyed up almost permanently and blood pressure may stay elevated. One way or another the body is harmed. The fight or flight response, as I said, has often been described. Less well known is its opposite, a later discovery, the 'relaxation response'.

The physiology of the relaxation response is decrease – in heart rate, blood pressure, breathing rate, oxygen consumption, metabolism, blood lactate, blood cortisone levels, brainwave frequency and muscle tension. Some of the decreases are extraordinary: oxygen consumption decreases to levels only found in very deep sleep or hibernating animals.

A detailed study of the relaxation response has been made by Dr Herbert Benson of the Harvard Medical School, in the USA. He studied the response in meditators, but in his book *The Relaxation Response* he gives a table of different techniques eliciting the physiologic changes of the relaxation response. These included various forms of Eastern meditation, progressive relaxation, autogenic training, and hypnosis with suggested deep relaxation. All of these relaxation methods will be described in this book. Readers are invited to experiment with methods and to find which methods relax them most.

The ability to relax and to take a relaxed and poised attitude to life – developed as an art when not innate – is essential for good health and for self-fulfilment. It means giving up the characteristic Western urge to be always up and doing and making an effort. Effort, it will be shown, is the thing to avoid for attaining a relaxed state. In contrast, wonders may be achieved by learning to 'let it happen' and to become at one with life's flow.


## BENEFITS

Reasons why you should learn to release tension from muscle and mind and to cultivate poised living will unfold as this book proceeds, but the following is a summary of the likely main benefits:

Improved health
Greater vitality
More energy in reserve, and a more economical and productive use of energy
Protection against stress, now a major killer, and from numerous psychosomatic disorders and diseases
Frequent elicitation of the relaxation response – which means a marked slowing down of physiological processes in the deep relaxation state. Increased alpha waves
Freedom from unnecessary tension
Protection for the heart and against high blood pressure
Improved digestion
Natural aid for all healing processes
Quicker onset of sleep and sleep of more refreshing quality
Poised posture in sitting, standing, walking, and all life's activities
Poised inner posture
Increased efficiency and economy of effort in work and play
Improved performance in arts and crafts, sports and games
Greater spontaneity in living
Feeling 'good' in the sense of good muscular and mental tone
Greater nervous stability and calmness
Reduced nervousness on important occasions
No dependence on tranquillizers or sleeping pills
Freedom from unrealistic fear and anxiety
Increased courage and confidence

Relaxed sense of humour

Enhanced sense of beauty

Purer perception and awareness

Feeling more fully alive

More harmonious relationships with parents, spouse, children, friends, neighbours, and workmates

Effortless concentration

Greater clarity of mind

More peace of mind

Increased creativity

Increased possibility of meaningful insights

Raised overall level of meaningfulness in living

Heightened awareness

Promotion of what the humanistic psychologists call self-actualization (growth towards full potential)

Integration of the personality

A diminution of dark, negative emotions and an increase of bright, positive emotions, such as generosity, optimism, joy, delight, love, compassion, and so on

Feeling of harmony with Nature and of following the natural order

Reacquaintance with the capacity – probably inoperative or rare since childhood or adolescence – of experiencing the pleasure and joy that there is in existence itself

More frequent peak experiences

Enhanced spiritual awareness and unfoldment

# 2 Progressive Relaxation

## WHAT IS PROGRESSIVE RELAXATION?

'Progressive relaxation' refers to all programmes of relaxation based on relaxing body muscles and muscle groups in sequence, usually concluding with mental relaxation. The method was established for use by an American doctor, Edmund Jacobson, who first began developing relaxation as a therapy in about 1910.

Dr Jacobson explored the subject scientifically. It was through his study of how to recognize tension and to let go from it that the word 'relaxation' came to be recognized as something other than its usual dictionary definition: remission of some constraint, duty, penalty, effort, etc., or recreation and amusement.

Progressive relaxation is now a well-established medical therapy, widely used by doctors and psychiatrists. The method is also familiar to many members of the general public, thanks to its appearance in popular books on coping with stress and 'nerves', and newspaper and magazine articles on the same subject.

When Dr Jacobson's *Progressive Relaxation* was published in 1929, it was described as 'a physiological and clinical investigation of muscular states and their significance in psychology and medical practice.' In medical practice Dr Jacobson had come to see how relaxation of the skeletal muscles could reduce wasteful expenditure of energy in patients 'not properly called neurotic' yet suffering unnecessarily from fatigue, debility and lowered resistance.

Because so many people pressed upon Dr Jacobson the value of describing his methods in ways assimilable to the general public, he wrote another book called *You Must Relax*, which was published in 1938, and revised and enlarged in 1976. The title is perhaps unfortunate, but this is the classic account of progressive relaxation of the body muscles, on which other methods are based.

Most psychotherapists using progressive relaxation today prefer to shorten the time given to each muscle group in the original method and to relax all body muscles at each session rather than take several days over each group. This is the modification I will employ here. The classic method allows for some adaptation, and the programmes given here are those I have personally found most direct and effective.

Because the training programme includes recognizing tension and letting go from it in all the main muscles and muscle groups, the programmes are set out step by step, which makes them look longer and more complicated than is in fact the case. Once you have gone through the procedure attentively a few times, you will find that the sequence is easily memorized and followed.

You will probably wish to experiment with other relaxation methods described in this book, but giving a few weeks to learning progressive relaxation will pay dividends. It has advantages over other methods and may also be combined with them effectively. The advantages are that no auto-suggestion or auto-hypnosis is involved, and no equipment, and that relaxation of body muscles as a neuromuscular skill based on direct body–mind rapport is not restricted solely to intensive sessions in which you lie or sit motionless, but may be used on numerous occasions in daily activity to relax muscles not needed for a particular action, thereby conserving energy, improving efficiency, and promoting psychophysical poise.

# RELAXATION AS A NEUROMUSCULAR SKILL

*Relaxing is letting go from tension in body and mind. Relaxation is the absence of unnecessary tension in body and mind*. It should not be confused with what usually passes as 'taking things easy for a few minutes'. This is considered to be effective relaxation if the body stays reasonably still for a short time and if the mind stays reasonably free from unpleasant thoughts or feelings. This is relaxation so far removed from its real possibilities as scarcely to warrant use of the name. The amount of refreshment and recuperation obtained is paltry compared with what may be experienced once relaxation is mastered as a neuromuscular skill. This sounds technical, but it simply means that mind and muscle learn to work together so that the mind's decision to let go from tension is obeyed.

That is what true relaxation is – a *letting go* from tension. Unfortunately most people have become so used to the presence of tension in their muscles that they are not aware of its being there except at times of severe stress. One has to be aware of tension before one can effectively let go from it. First awareness. Then letting go. A neuromuscular skill.

Don't let the words 'neuromuscular skill' worry you. Whoever you are, you have learned scores of neuromuscular skills in your time. Standing and walking, running and jumping, kicking or throwing a ball – these are all neuromuscular skills; so are brushing your teeth or hair, putting on socks, and buttoning a jacket. And just as all these skills can be performed well or badly, so we will be concerned in this book with relaxing body and mind effectively.

Quality rest for body and mind can be cultivated as yet another skill among the many you now possess. And what a beneficial skill to have!

The preparatory training in progressive relaxation is enjoyable and rewarding in itself. It is easily understood. It can be taught to young children, and studied and learned for themselves by older children. There is no grasping after elusive abstractions and the techniques involve simple acts of awareness. If there is any difficulty at first, it will be the utter simplicity of what is required. Total relaxation is achieved by progressive stages, going over the whole body from toes to head while letting go from tension.

## THE TWO PROGRAMMES

Programme One is a conditioning programme. Its aim is to enable you to recognize tension in the main muscles and muscle groups of the body, and also in the muscles responsible for thought. It is easily overlooked that there are muscles of thought; they are the muscles which move and focus the eyes and those which are used for speech. Imagery and silent speech are the basis of thinking. We are aware of the imagery, but it takes sensitive electrical equipment to point out that in thinking we go in for subtle talking. Stay with Programme One for a month, then use Programme Two.

In Programme Two tension is not deliberately induced. As through the earlier conditioning programme you will have learned to recognize even low amounts of tension, you now go over the same muscles in the same sequence and let go again. By then you should be able to know the feeling both of tension and of relaxation. The sequence of muscle relaxation has also been memorized and should present no difficulty.

You may find that you wish to continue with Programme One even though you have practised it daily for a month. You could have two relaxation sessions a day, each of about twenty minutes. You could use Programme One in the morning when awareness is sharp and use Programme Two in the evening.

Even if you feel that you have learned to recognize tension and to let go from it through the conditioning programme, it is helpful to occasionally use it as a kind of 'refresher course'.

After some months of training you may be able to let go from tension rapidly by moving your attention swiftly over the whole body or giving attention only to the arms, legs and face muscles. But that technique is for use only when time is strictly limited, or in emergencies.

The programmes are described for a person lying on his or her

back, but after two or three months' training they should also
be used when sitting. This increases the opportunities for using
the technique.

## MAKE FRIENDS WITH YOUR MUSCLES

Success in progressive relaxation is attained by a method of
muscle control and communication. This could be called
'getting on good speaking terms with your muscles'. To do
this you don't require the muscular development of a Mr or a
Miss Universe: any man, woman or child has muscles that come
under voluntary control, and by making friends with them they
will relax at the asking. You ask your left leg to relax and it
relaxes. You ask your right arm to relax and it relaxes. You ask
your jaw to relax and it relaxes.

This is achieved by first learning to be aware of tension in
twenty-four muscles and muscle groups, which are relaxed in
sequence, moving up from the feet to the forehead and scalp.
Even the thinking muscles will be relaxed.

Here are the twenty-four muscles and muscle groups:

1  Feet
2  Lower legs (front)
3  Lower legs (rear)
4  Upper legs (front)
5  Upper legs (rear)
6  Buttocks
7  Abdomen
8  Lower back
9  Upper back
10  Breasts (pectorals)
11  Hands
12  Forearms
13  Upper arms (front)
14  Upper arms (rear)
15  Shoulders
16  Diaphragm and thorax
17  Trapezius (across base of neck)

18  Neck
19  Throat
20  Jaw
21  Lips
22  Tongue
23  Eyes
24  Forehead and scalp

The twenty-four body parts are learned in sequence during the actual training – but run your eyes down the list a few times now. Be aware of each part of the body as you name it.

Conditioning in progressive relaxation consists of contracting the muscles in sequence and taking note of the sensation of tension. Each week, after the first of the four weeks given to Programme One, reduce the intensity of the muscle contractions so that you are having to be aware of progressively fainter amounts of tension. It is just as important to note the feeling of relaxation as you let go from tension.

In theory, muscular relaxation seems the simplest of attainments. It is doing nothing. You allow nothing to happen in your muscles. It is a sad commentary on the nature of life today that doing nothing is so difficult for so many people.

What is felt when letting go is followed right through is real relaxation. It is found to be very different from what had previously been looked upon as relaxation.

## PROGRAMME ONE

Relaxation should take place in a quiet, softly lit room that is pleasantly warm, airy but free from draughts. Later you may be able to relax even with slight discomfort or distraction, but the most favourable conditions are best sought in the first months of training.

Lie on your back on a comfortable, though not too yielding surface: a bed, divan or couch – or on the floor, softened by a folded rug or blanket. Too hard a surface causes discomfort; too yielding a surface creates muscle tensions.

Distractions and disturbances of all kinds should be reduced to the unavoidable minimum when relaxing. Empty your bladder before lying down to relax; bowel also if a possible source of distraction.

It is helpful in early training if the room in which you practise relaxation is pleasant, with pleasant associations. Unpleasant associations can produce tensions. A man who had read one of my books about relaxation wrote telling me of his difficulties: only when on holiday could he attain refreshing relaxation on lying down and letting go. He was baffled by it. He wrote again some months later to say he had located the trouble: a photograph which showed the correspondent with a fine crop of curly hair – alas, long since reaped by merciless Time! Once the picture had been removed from the room, progress in relaxation was made.

## The relaxation position

Having established the best conditions for relaxation, adopt the relaxation position.

Lie flat on your back, with your body fully supported from heels to head. Lying down, freeing yourself from gravity's drag, is essential for full relaxation. When lying down comfortably it is easy to give full attention to relaxing your muscles.

Lie full length on your back. Rest your arms, slightly bent at the elbows, alongside your body and a little out from it, the palms of your hands down, your fingers spread a little apart. Your hand should feel loose, like a glove.

Your legs should be extended, but not locked at the knees, kept a little apart, and the feet relaxed and falling out a little to each side.

The backs of the head and neck, the lower back and the under thighs may be supported by thin cushions, care being taken that the shoulders and hips are not cushioned. If your posture is poor and your lower back does not settle down on the surface on which you lie, without a cushion against the lumbar region you may feel tension in the lower back and deep in the abdomen. The problem is the tightening of the *psoas*, a rather strange

...uscle which runs through the abdomen from the small of the back to the tops of the thigh bones.

Your clothing should be loose and comfortable.

Once settled in the relaxation position, you are ready to commence the conditioning controls. Eventually you will be able to recognize even faint traces of tension in a muscle apparently at rest.

Hold each contraction about six seconds. Be fully aware of the sensations in the contracted muscles. Be as fully aware of the sensations of relaxation when you let go from the contractions.

## Stretch

First you lie down on your back, body fully supported.

Then you STRETCH.

Stretch as a cat stretches . . . smoothly, slowly, lingeringly, luxuriating in it. Do you know of a better model for relaxation both in repose and in action than the cat? When more than two thousand years ago the Yogins of India devised their system of body–mind relaxation and integration, they based it on the stretching actions and postures they observed in jungle cats.

Straighten your arms, raise them parallel overhead, then stretch them as far beyond your head as they will go. Reach out with your fingertips.

At the same time stretch your legs away from you, sliding your heels along the bed or floor and pointing your toes.

Breathe out in a long sigh as you stretch both your arms and your legs in opposite directions for about ten seconds. Enjoy every second of the stretch, feeling tension dissolving in the muscles.

Then bring your arms back to the relaxation position and *let go.*

## Close your eyes

As you let go with all of yourself, close your eyes. This is another essential for learning relaxation. Closing the eyes cuts off the bombardment of visual stimuli on the retina, with the mental associations so many of them trigger in chain reaction.

And behind the lowered lids the attention is more easily mobilized to act like a torch beam moving from muscle to muscle.

Attention quietly collected to focus like a torch beam in a dark room, direct it as follows. . . .

## Rhythmical breathing

Observe your breathing. Which means, as your eyes are closed, that you become aware of your breathing in those places where air impinges on the sensitive lining of the nostrils and in the muscular rise and fall of the abdomen which accompanies relaxed breathing, together with some expansion and contraction of the lower ribs.

For two or three minutes simply be aware of your breathing, and of its rhythm. Then easefully slow down your rate of breathing by slightly lengthening your inhalations and lengthening your exhalations rather more. Don't cram air into your lungs; keep your breathing comfortable. The longer exhalations release tension – a slow, smooth letting out of air, rather like a heartfelt sigh.

After breathing in this quiet rhythmical way for about three minutes, you are ready to start the toes-to-scalp conditioning sequence.

## Conditioning controls

A few points about the tense-and-let-go controls are worth making again.

Without forcing concentration, be passively aware in each control of the sensations of contraction and the subsequent sensations of relaxation as you let go from tension. Being aware of the tension gives you something to let go from.

Again it is necessary to remind the reader that you will not relax by trying. Letting it happen is the key. Let go from tension and relaxation happens. You passively observe it as it happens. The muscles will flop of their own accord.

## Feet

We commence our toes to head relaxation controls at our lower extremities.

Tense and nervous people betray their condition with agitated movements of the hands and feet. They tap their feet, press them together, stab their toes against the floor, curl their toes or press them back against the foot; curl a foot around an ankle, calf or chair leg; twist a foot first to one side and then to the other side; press down weightily with their feet as though trying to take root in the ground. Be on guard against unnecessary tensions in the feet. Here is how to train yourself to recognize them.

*Right foot (top)*: Focus your attention on your right foot. Without moving the rest of the foot, bend up the toes. You will experience sensations of tension in the upper surface of the foot. Give full attention to these sensations for about six seconds, then let go, taking note for about the same duration of the sensation of relaxation in the top of the foot.

*Right foot (sole)*: Now, again without moving the rest of the foot, curl your toes in strongly towards the sole of the foot. This time the tension lines will traverse the sole of the foot. Be aware. Let go with the toes so that they spring back to their normal alignment with the foot. Be aware now of the relaxation in the foot.

*Left foot (top and sole)*: Repeat the toe-raising and toe-curling controls with your other foot, concentrating again on tension and on relaxation in the upper and lower foot.

Reverse the right-left feet and legs sequence if you tend to kick a ball with your left foot.

## Lower legs

*Right lower leg (front)*: Keeping the rest of the leg steady, bend up the whole right foot against the ankle joint. This time you will feel the contraction in the front of the lower leg from ankle to knee. Let go from it.

*Right lower leg (rear)*: Now point the toes of your right foot strongly away from you, contracting the calf muscle at the rear of the lower leg. Sustain the contraction, then let go from it.

*Left lower leg (front and rear)*: With your left foot, repeat the controls just described, contracting and relaxing the lower leg, front and rear, with full awareness.

The foregoing controls will have demonstrated to you how tense people add to their problem when they make the bending and twisting movements of the feet referred to earlier. Foot movements contract the muscles and tendons of the lower leg and build up muscular tensions that send back messages to the brain, augmenting the anxiety state that produced the restlessness in the first place.

## Upper legs

Sitting awkwardly, crossing the legs, squeezing the legs together – these contribute to tensions in the upper legs. People who stand for long periods in their jobs or professions, often awkwardly, such as dentists and shop assistants, are prone to leg aches and pains, swellings and distended veins. Such people should take a leaf out of the Yogin's book and rest frequently with the feet on a higher level than the body, reversing the normal pull of gravity on the legs.

*Right upper leg (front)*: Draw up your right knee a little, pulling the heel back towards you a few inches. Immediately slide your heel away from you and straighten the leg fully, locking it at the knee. The powerful front thigh muscles will contract. Hold the contraction, then let go from it and let the leg go limp. Note the feeling of relaxation.

*Right upper leg (rear)*: Shift your attention to the *biceps* at the back of the thigh which flex the leg. Contract it now by drawing the knee up a few inches, bending the leg, and pressing the heel down and back. As the attempt is made and blocked to flex the leg, the *biceps* of the thigh will contract. Observe the static (isometric) contraction produced, and the relaxation when you let go and return the leg to a resting position.

*Left upper legs (front and rear)*: Repeat the controls for contracting and relaxing the right upper leg, front and back, this time with the left leg.

## Buttocks

The twin buttock muscles can be contracted and relaxed by stretching your legs away from you and tilting the pelvis forward, assisting with mental control. There should be no difficulty in feeling the contraction and in letting go from it.

## Abdomen

When we consider that the abdomen houses the important gathering of nerves called the solar plexus, and that it acts as a muscular corset supporting and protecting such vital visceral organs as the stomach, liver, spleen, pancreas, kidneys, intestines and transverse colon, we can appreciate why tension so often seizes us in this middle region of the body when we are under pressure. The sensation so tellingly described as 'having butterflies in the stomach' is one example of experiencing nervous tension in the abdomen.

This area of the body is the first to become flabby when we fail to take sufficient exercise, with the result that the visceral organs lack proper support and protection. Time spent in toning and firming the abdominal muscles is time well spent. So is time given to learning to release tension from these muscles.

The abdominal muscles are intimately connected with the act of breathing, so that tension in these muscles hampers breathing. Fortunately the converse applies: by relaxing the abdomen, respiratory activity is set free from tension.

In Japan the region around the navel is known as *hara* and it is given a significance far beyond anything accorded to it in the West. See chapter 7.

To contract the abdominal muscles: bring your shoulders up and forwards as though going to sit up, tensing the abdominal wall without actually lifting the centre of your back from its support. With a little practice you will find that you can make the abdomen very firm. Mind–muscle control contributes. Observe this tautness for six seconds, then let go from it and observe the result for about ten seconds.

Dr Jacobson and some other writers on progressive relaxation recommend drawing in the stomach muscles as a conditioning control. However, my studies in physical culture, yoga, etc., have shown that the abdomen may be fully relaxed when drawn in. If the lungs have been emptied of air and the abdomen is kept relaxed, the abdominal wall will actually be drawn back involuntarily into the thoracic cavity. One could contract the abdominal muscles by pulling back on full lungs, but that would not be a desirable practice. I prefer the contraction of the abdominal wall described in the preceding paragraph.

### Back

*Lower Back*: For many people, tension causes aches and pains in the muscles of the lower back, often given the general name of lumbago. Other causes of back complaints are poor posture and equally poor design in chairs. This is a key stress area.

Now create tension in the lower back by arching the spine. As soon as you do this you will experience a wave of muscular tightness across the small of the back. Give your full attention to this uncomfortable feeling for six seconds, then let go, lowering the backbone to its former resting position.

*Upper back (shoulder blades)*: Draw your shoulders back and in as though to meet behind you, folding in the broad 'wings' of muscle covering the shoulderblades. Hold the contraction, note the sensations, let go, note the feeling of reduced tension.

*Breasts (pectorals)*

These muscles draw the arms inwards. The pectorals underlie the fatty breasts in a woman and support them. We can make the pectorals contract by pressing in with the hands against the upper thighs. Observe the sensations of bunching in the chest muscles and the contrasting relaxation as the pressure is lifted.

*Hands*

Though a right-left sequence is given for the hands and arms, left-handed people should reverse this order and commence with the left hand.

*Right hand*: (a) With the palm of your hand flat down, bend your fingers up and back. The heel of your hand and the palm stay firmly in place. The fingers will not lift more than an inch or two, but this will be enough to contract the back of the hand.

(b) Make a fist of the hand and squeeze tightly. This will contract the inside of the hand. Tension will also be felt in the fingers and in the forearm.

*Left hand*: Repeat the (a) and (b) contractions with the left hand.

The hands are another key centre for relaxation. Their significance is shown when we clench them in moments of stress. The most important areas for relaxation, links in the chain of body–mind tension, are the face, the hands, the lower back and the muscles of breathing.

*Arms*

*Right forearm*: Palm down, raise the whole hand up and back against the wrist joint. Forearm and wrist stay down, all of the hand comes up. You will feel lines of tension running up the forearm. Let the hand go limp and note the relaxation in the forearm.

*Left forearm*: Now take note of the tension that results in the left forearm as you raise your left hand up and back against the wrist.

*Right upper arm (front)*: Turn upward the palm of your right hand. Keeping your upper arm steady, flex your arm and bring up your hand until the fingers touch or almost touch your right shoulder. This will contract the biceps muscle on the inside of the upper arm, whose chief function is to flex the arm. Contract, then return the arm to its resting position.

*Right upper arm (rear)*: Our starting position this time is the position of arm flexion adopted in the preceding control, with fingers touching or almost touching the right shoulder. Now slowly extend the arm until it is fully straightened, which is accomplished by the triceps muscle to the rear of the upper arm. Contract, keeping the arm 'locked', then let go, bending the arm slightly again in the resting position.

*Left upper arm (front)*: Contract the biceps of the left arm by flexing the arm.

*Left upper arm (rear)*: From the position of arm flexion, slowly straighten the arm and sustain the contraction for about six seconds before letting go fully.

## Shoulders

A frequent sign of tension is a person holding the shoulders too high. They hang loosely when a person is relaxed.

*Right shoulder*: Straighten the right arm and slowly raise it to a vertical position, concentrating on the pull from the right shoulder. Lower the arm to the starting position and relax the arm.

*Left shoulder*: Contract the muscles of the left shoulder by raising the straightened left arm.

*Diaphragm and thorax*

Breathe in slowly and deeply, though not so deeply that you feel strained. Feel the diaphragm lower and the intercostal muscles separate the ribs as the lungs inflate. The image of an umbrella being opened and closed comes to mind. As you fill your lungs and hold the inhalation for a few seconds, take careful note of all muscular tensions. And again as you empty the lungs. A full exhalation, a real letting go, is essential to relaxed breathing; in its turn, relaxed breathing promotes health and general relaxation. Unless there is a blockage, breathe in and out through the nostrils.

This control, correctly performed several times, takes away feelings of constriction in the chest and diaphragm, and encourages correct breathing habits that will fortify bodily health in years to come.

Perform three complete inhalations and exhalations, really letting go on the latter. Let tensions flow out with the breath.

*Trapezius, neck, throat*

*Trapezius*: These muscles lie across the top of the back, against the base of the neck and to each of its sides. They are contracted by shrugging your shoulders. Hold the contraction, then let go.

*Neck*: Press back your head, thus contracting the rear neck muscles. Sustain the contraction for six seconds before relaxing the muscles. Now bend your head to the right, tensing the right side of the neck. Resume the vertical head position, then bend your head to the left, contracting the left side of the neck. Each tilt of the head provides a contraction for the attention to dwell on. Don't confuse the stretching feeling on the opposite side of the neck to which you bend the head with the contraction of the neck muscles that tilts the head.

*Throat*: Recognize and memorize tensions in the muscles of the throat by pressing your chin down firmly on to your chest. Pay attention to the contraction, then bring your chin back to level.

*Face and scalp*

Having established some degree of rapport with every main muscle or muscle group from your feet up to your neck and throat, you should go on to do the same with the face and scalp.

The muscles of the face are the most important of all we have sought to control, for their relaxation provides the key to relaxing the mind itself.

The muscles of the face are the most subtle and extraordinary we possess, combining strength and delicacy to a unique degree. No other group of emotions we have responds so sensitively to the play of the emotions – one of the reasons why they have such an important part to play in attaining real relaxation. The other reason is that they provide the key to relaxing the *mind*.

The face muscles respond to exercise like any other muscles: a few simple exercises can influence their shape, firmness, tone and suppleness. My book on exercising the facial muscles, *New Faces*, contains exercises of the kind now to be employed for gaining control over the face muscles.

*Jaw*: Clench your jaw by bringing your upper and lower teeth firmly together, though not so firmly as to risk shattering your molars. Be aware of the sensations of contraction in the jaw muscles, then let go fully from tension so that the jaw loosens and the teeth part.

*Lips*: Press your lips together firmly as though in strong disapproval of something. Sustain the pressure, then let the lips go loose.

*Tongue*: Keeping your upper and lower teeth lightly together, curl up your tongue and press it up and back against the roof of your mouth. Feel the contraction of the tongue as it pushes upwards. After six seconds, let your tongue rest flat in the bottom of your mouth with the tip behind the lower teeth.

*Eyes*: Six small muscles move the eyeballs. Few people have ever given a thought to relaxing them. They often go on working busily in sleep, following the movements of the figures in dreams just as they would in waking life.

You can get to know tension in the eyeball muscles by looking as far to the right as possible without moving your head, then as far to the left, as far above, as far below. In terms of a clock face, this would mean looking three o'clock, nine o'clock, twelve o'clock, and six o'clock. At each limit of the eyes' movement, hold the contraction for about six seconds.

There is a further way to recognize tension in the eye muscles. Stare hard at something for six seconds. Be aware of the sensations of tension in and around the eyes. Staring creates tension without helping the eyesight. Let go and blink a few times, then close the eyes and rest them for a few seconds before moving on to the next control.

*Forehead and scalp*: What I want you to do now is frown fiercely, drawing in and tensing the muscles of the forehead. At the same time the frown will tug at the scalp due to the action of the *occipito frontalis* muscle which starts above the eyebrows and extends beneath the scalp over the top of the head to the back of the skull. When this muscle tightens, it feels as though a steel band is tightening around the head. Relaxation therapists teach sufferers from tension headaches (migraine) to relax this large muscle. This exercise can be used to combat worry.

After frowning hard, relax the whole face, letting it widen, helped by a smile.

## THE MIND-CALMING TECHNIQUE

It is essential to mastery of this technique that you learn to detect degrees of tension in the visual and speech muscles. Give your full attention to these tensions and to the contrasting sensations of relaxation when you *let go*. As most of your thinking is through visual imagery and inward speaking, control over the visual and speech muscles is the key to bringing peace to the mind.

## Part 1.  *Visual*

For this exercise in visualization, choose a favourite restful scene or picture from the store of them in your memory. With eyes still closed, project before your mind's eye as clear and detailed a picture as possible. Let your eyes roam easily over the scene. Mark the slight tension in the eyes during visualization. Now *let go* with your visual muscles and note how the tension dwindles and simultaneously the picture fades and darkens. The more you relax your visual muscles the deeper will be the blackness before your eyes. Really *let go*.

Do it again. The scene before the mind's eye, bright and clear. Start letting go with the visual muscles. Fade out the picture into blackness, the blacker the better.

## Part 2.  *Speech*

You now use your speech muscles and take note of the dwindling of tension as you lower your voice, aware also that tension still exists when you merely think a sentence.

Say aloud: 'I am bringing peace to my mind.' Note the tension in your speech muscles. Repeat the sentence more softly. More softly again. Whisper it. Say it subvocally. Finally, think it. Note the progressive lessening of tension, but that it still exists faintly when you think in words.

Perform the control again. Aloud: 'I am bringing peace to my mind.' More softly. More softly again. Whisper it. Say it soundlessly, looking for tension in the speech muscles. Think: 'I am bringing peace to my mind.'

Now *let go* with your speech muscles from the tension in them you have experienced, strong at first, then fainter as you whispered, spoke subvocally, and finally as you thought the sentence. Be aware of how the mind quietens as you let go.

Your lips should be lightly together, your teeth just parted, your jaw muscles and throat muscles at ease, your tongue flat and broad in your mouth with its tip behind the lower teeth. Let all tension go from these speech muscles. Let them fully relax.

## PROGRAMME TWO

Make yourself fully comfortable in the relaxation position. Let your gaze wander easily for a few seconds, then close your eyes.

Direct your attention to your breathing. Let it be slow, smooth and rhythmical. Breathe through the nostrils, deep into your abdomen, but without cramming the lungs. Breathe gently, smoothly and easily.

By now, through use of Programme One once or twice daily for a month, you should have conditioned yourself to recognize tension and to let go from it in the chief muscles and muscle groups of your body. Now you let go from tension merely by being aware of the muscles without deliberately contracting them. Move your attention over your body as lightly as a torch beam. Really *let go*, relaxing with your full weight.

The sequence is as before. By now you should be easily familiar with it.

Focus your attention gently like a torch beam on each body part in turn, searching for signs of tension. Take three or four seconds on this, then *let go fully* with the body part so that all tension drains away and the muscles feel loose and limp and resting with their full weight. Be aware of relaxation for about ten seconds. You lie motionless, breathing easily and gently. The programme is carried out in *awareness*.

Here is the sequence again:

Right foot (top)
Right foot (sole)
Left foot (top)
Left foot (sole)
Right lower leg (front)
Right lower leg (rear)
Left lower leg (front)
Left lower leg (rear)
Right upper leg (front)
Right upper leg (rear)
Left upper leg (front)
Left upper leg (rear)

(If you tend to kick a ball with your left foot, start the preceding controls with your left foot and then the right foot, reversing the order given here.)

Buttocks
Abdomen
Lower back
Upper back (shoulder blades)
Breasts (pectorals)
(Start below with your predominant hand)
Right hand
Left hand
Right forearm
Left forearm
Right upper arm (front)
Right upper arm (rear)
Left upper arm (front)
Left upper arm (rear)
Right shoulder
Left shoulder
Diaphragm and thorax
Trapezius
Neck
Throat
Jaw
Lips
Tongue
Eyes
Forehead and scalp
Let go with your visual muscles. See blackness
Let go with your speech muscles: throat, jaw, tongue, etc
Let go and bring peace to the mind

Sustain the bodily relaxation and mental calm. If thoughts intrude of other than a relaxing nature, relax your visual and speech muscles again, or go over the full programme.

# CONCISE KEY TO THE CONDITIONING
# MOVEMENTS

| No. | To contract the | Movement |
|-----|-----------------|----------|
| 1 | foot | bend up toes |
| 2 | lower leg (front) | bend up foot |
| 3 | lower leg (rear) | point toes |
| 4 | upper leg (front) | bend then straighten leg |
| 5 | upper leg (rear) | pull heel back |
| 6 | buttocks | stretch legs |
| 7 | abdomen | tense abdominal wall |
| 8 | lower back | arch spine |
| 9 | upper back | shoulders back and in |
| 10 | breasts (pectorals) | hands in against thighs |
| 11 | hand | bend up fingers |
|  |  | make tight fist |
| 12 | forearm | bend up hand |
| 13 | upper arm (front) | flex arm |
| 14 | upper arm (rear) | straighten arm |
| 15 | shoulder | raise straight arm |
| 16 | diaphragm and thorax | deep breath and hold |
| 17 | trapezius | shrug shoulders |
| 18 | neck | press back head |
| 19 | throat | press chin on to chest |
| 20 | jaw | clench teeth |
| 21 | lips | press lips together |
| 22 | tongue | teeth together, press tongue against roof of mouth |
| 23 | eyes | look right, left, up, down |
| 24 | forehead and scalp | frown |
| 25 | thinking muscles | visualize scene, think verbally |

# PROGRESSIVE RELAXATION THERAPY

The chapter headings in *You Must Relax* indicate the diseases and disorders that Dr Jacobson found beneficially influenced by progressive relaxation – nervous disorders, high blood pressure, heart strain and coronary troubles, insomnia, indigestion and colitis. Within the chapters one finds discussion of angina, arthritis, bowel movements as a sign of tension, breathing under tension, overstimulated children, colic, eye tension, fatigue, fear, fever, glands, grey hair, headache, hypochondria, hysteria, infection, intestines, nervous breakdown, neuroses, pain relief, phobias, pituitary gland, psychiatric disorders, skin disorders, spastic colon, spastic digestive tract, spastic oesophagus, stammering, stomach ulcers, and worry – in all of these relaxation therapy is appropriate.

Dr Jacobson established the relationship between muscle tension and the workings of the mind. He showed that anxiety and deep muscular relaxation cannot exist together.

He also showed that learned relaxation of the skeletal muscles can extend to smooth involuntary muscle in the body. Relaxation training can thus influence the cardiovascular and gastrointestinal systems.

Progressive relaxation is often used today in the psychiatric treatment of phobias by desensitization. In this treatment the patient learns to relax when confronted by the situation in which fear is aroused. Gradually relaxation conquers the fear.

Progressive relaxation methods are often used also in biofeedback therapy for stress-related disorders. Once skill is acquired in recognizing tension in the skeletal muscles and in letting go from it, progressive relaxation may be usefully combined with any other relaxation method and therapy.

# 3 Relaxation in Action

This topic has been introduced at a stage when you can only begin to apply the lessons learned from starting training in one form of psycho-physical relaxation – progressive relaxation. But it is important to make an early start in bringing relaxation into day-to-day activities – producing poise – and training in progressive relaxation equips you well for this aim.

Programme One and Programme Two in the preceding chapter induce *general* relaxation, but the method used was *progressive* relaxation of body parts – hand, forearm, upper arm, and so on. Total relaxation is attained by means of *specific* relaxation, letting go from tension in particular muscles and muscle groups. It is this aspect of progressive relaxation that is so useful in applying muscular relaxation in daily activities. You acquire skill in recognizing and in letting go from unnecessary tension – in standing, sitting, walking, running, doing housework, typing, driving a car, playing golf, speaking, looking, hearing, and even in thinking.

## DIFFERENTIAL RELAXATION

Specific tension and specific relaxation work together to carry out physical activity. One muscle group contracts while its antagonist group relaxes; there is shortening of muscle and there is lengthening of muscle. When the biceps muscle of the upper arm contracts to flex the arm, the triceps lengthens. When the triceps contracts to straighten the arm, the biceps lets go. Each muscle group has its turn to tense and its turn to relax according to the action required.

Training in progressive relaxation gives you control over specific tension and relaxation. Applying this in daily activity, you can learn to let some muscles relax while others contract. Physical poise is attained when only muscles essential for any task are contracted to the minimum extent required for optimal efficiency and all other muscles are relaxed. Dr Edmund Jacobson called this 'differential relaxation'. The resulting activity looks and feels natural, balanced and 'right' – as one sees in the instinctive movements of animals. Hence one can speak of relaxation in action, or poised action.

Total relaxation in action is not possible. If you tried it when standing still, you would collapse in a heap on the floor. Like the falling drunk man, you would probably not be injured, because you were relaxed when you fell. But a balance of relaxation and minimum contraction is needed for those times when you are not lying fully supported, which is the only occasion when general relaxation is possible. Differential relaxation should then be applied: in early training in relaxed living the application will often be conscious, but eventually it will become habitual and your movements will flow as if from a calm centre.

Differential relaxation saves energy and wear and tear. It is the hallmark of the skilled performer in every art, craft and sport. Outer poise is admired in the Orient because of what it reveals about the inner posture or being of a person. That aspect of relaxation in action will be discussed later in this book.

Dr Jacobson found it desirable to train patients in differential as well as in general relaxation, because patients overactive and overaroused in daily life found it difficult to let go on lying down to relax, as they usually did on lying down to be still and go to sleep.

A useful beginning in learning differential relaxation is to apply its principles to how you sit.

## SITTING RELAXED

The best kind of chair to sit in for starting learning relaxed sitting is one that supports your bottom, back and head. Later you can apply the technique while sitting in other types of chair. Keep your legs a little apart and both feet flat on the floor. Crossing ankles or legs sets up tensions and impedes circulation. Locking ankles beneath a chair or tucking toes behind a calf muscle is nearly always a sign of tension in a sitter. Support your hands on the arms of the chair or in your lap. The neck should be relaxed and the head and back should be in alignment; when leaning forward to stand up or to sit down, jack-knife from the pelvis. Lead with your head in rising from a chair, your torso following. (See chapter 7, which describes poised posture.)

In a sitting posture the procedure for learning relaxation is not much different from that for lying down. Using Programme One and Programme Two will give you experiential knowledge of the degree of relaxation possible when sitting. Slight adaptation may be made in some of the tense-and-let-go controls. For example, to contract the pectoral muscles you could press in on the arms of the chair rather than on the thighs. If you sit with your bottom, back and head supported, the controls may all be performed as given in the preceding chapter with only minor adaptation if any. Shift awareness up the body in the same sequence from feet to scalp, with similar timing. Look on this as training performed in addition to general relaxation lying down.

When skill is developed in relaxation sitting in a chair, the feeling of relaxation can be carried into standing and moving postures for some time after rising from the chair.

## READING

Differential relaxation may be practised while sitting and reading. The body is relaxed as far as possible. Your hands and arms are given sufficient strength to hold the book, though use of a book rest may be considered. Look at the book and read a few lines. Now start to let go with the muscles of the eyes and forehead. Many people are surprised to find that they cannot then read the words. They may be aware vaguely of the print, but not of the meaning of the words. Next increase the tension slightly until you just reach the point where the words can be read. You will find that reading at this pressure, without loss of meaning, is easiest on the eyes.

Another way to fade out the meaning of print before your eyes is to relax the speech muscles, checking the subvocalization that goes on in reading. Some people move their lips while reading. This relaxation cures the habit.

## WRITING

Students and people who write with pen or pencil for a considerable time each day will benefit from experimenting to find the easiest posture, which is head poised in line with back, for this activity, and the minimum pressure needed to actually use the pen or pencil. If you lean forward over a desk or table, tilt from the pelvis not the waist or the neck. Rest your free arm on the desk or table or in your lap. The saving in energy from such practical adjustments is not inconsiderable and physical fatigue is less likely to impair mental powers. By the way, some people find that their handwriting improves after training in relaxation.

When writing or typing for long periods, it is helpful to occasionally relax the neck muscles and rotate the head slowly in a clockwise and then in an anti-clockwise direction.

## BENDING, LIFTING, CARRYING

Here again the main thing to remember to reduce strain on the spine is to bend from the hip joints and not from the waist or the neck. Bending forward from the waist rounds the spine and makes it vulnerable to injury in thc lower vertebrae, particularly when you are lifting something. Bending the head forward from the neck imposes a strain on the top vertebrae, where the spine comes up to the skull.

By squatting down with feet apart to pick up a low object, the poised alignment of head, neck and back can be maintained to give the best position of leverage and the best posture for protection against injury.

When carrying a heavy object, hold it against your body, reducing the load on the spine.

## ACQUIRING PHYSICAL SKILLS

Physical skills of all kinds depend on differential relaxation for efficiency and economy of effort. The principle can be applied to any human activity. It makes gardening, housework, dressing, washing, shaving, cooking, and so on less energy consuming, more efficient and more pleasant because more poised.

Arts, crafts, sports and games all depend on the correct use of specific relaxation for success.

## POISED PERFORMANCE

The true 'professionals' in occupations and sports display physical poise in performance. They show economy of movement and effort. To watch them perform is a pleasure. They give the appearance of making what they do look easy. The great footballer, cricketer or tennis player is often described as 'making time', 'creating space' and 'making the ball do the work'. Grace and poise come through training, but an essential part of that training is using only the muscles essential to performance and relaxing the others.

Rhythm and timing have prominent roles in poised performance. The skilled craftsman demonstrates these qualities as well as the dancer or the boxer.

Men and women engaged in 'back breaking' labour will sing in unison, thereby inducing rhythm into their physical movements. Work songs are an important part of folk music.

The restraints and distortions of the 'civilized' way of life destroy our natural rhythms. One way to destroy natural rhythm that the 'professional' knows about is to press too hard, to force beyond a certain point. When it comes to the crucial putt, the pot black that wins a snooker game, the final game of the last set in tennis, then what is needed is all the player's relaxation, poise, awareness and effortless use of muscles accompanied by a bright but calm alertness. Champions have these qualities.

One definition of rhythm given in the *Oxford Dictionary* is 'due correlation and interdependence of parts, producing a harmonious whole'. This definition would also apply to poised performance.

Along with instinctive or trained balanced use of the body muscles, of their contraction and expansion, goes breathing harmonized to the muscular action. Breathing rhythms are a key factor in promoting relaxed and poised living.

It is worth mentioning that having the end result in mind while performing a physical action may often be a recipe for disaster. It is better to concentrate on what has to be done, step by step. Focusing attention on means rather than ends was an interesting teaching of F. Matthias Alexander, who originated a method of postural training that we will be describing later.

For some years I collected newspaper and magazine cuttings and typed notes of material in books on the part relaxation plays in training a person to sing, to play the violin or piano, to swim, and so on. Eventually, when three card files were bulging with notes and cuttings, I called a halt to collecting, with proof that differential relaxation is at the heart of skill in numerous human activities based on body use.

Professional singers learn to make full use of their breath and vocal cords through combining relaxation with control of breathing from the diaphragm. The throat and jaw muscles are relaxed as much as possible. The least tension in the jaw muscles starts a trembling in the jaw and turns the singing into a sheep's bleat.

When a voice is perfectly 'placed' it does not have to be *robusto* to carry easily to the back row of an opera house even on soft head notes. John McCormack and Chaliapin were renowned for this. Chaliapin said he liked to sing very softly because it made his audience hold their breath and concentrate intently on his singing.

## EXERCISE SYSTEMS

When it comes to exercise systems, the two most associated with relaxation are Yoga postures and Tai chi ch'uan. So much depends on how one performs movement exercises. Swimming is relaxing when well within strength capacity. Being in water effectively reduces bodyweight relative to exercising in air. Some years ago a man called Togna devised an exercise system for use while having a bath. The fact that movements are so much easier in water than out of it is the basis of therapy for spastics and other people with movement difficulties.

Yoga does not involve active exercise. A few, but not many, of the postures require great muscle effort; they are those that most resemble Western gymnastic exercises. Most Yoga *asanas* are static postures, held motionless with many muscles relaxed. One asana is called the 'corpse posture' – in it you lie on your back as though dead, letting relaxation happen.

Tai ch'i chuan are Chinese slow-motion exercises. The movements harmonize body use and breathing and have a mind relaxing contemplative effect. Though illustrated books of instruction are available, this exercise system is difficult to learn from the printed page and classes are not easy to find.

Some held Yoga postures require static or isometric muscle contractions. *Isometrics* is the name of a system of static muscle contraction exercises that were developed in the USA in the 1960s. This type of muscle contraction makes an excellent preparation for becoming familiar with tension in body muscles. A movement (isotonic) exercise is attempted but blocked by an unyielding resistance that can be a heavy piece of furniture or one's own body. Pressing, pushing, pulling or squeezing in against the immovable object produces specific muscle tension. If using the method to learn to relax, the strength of the contractions should be gradually diminished until very faint and produced by only slight pressure. Take three or four weeks to reach that point, starting with contractions at about two thirds of your maximum strength. Programmes for all the main body muscles and muscle groups from feet to face may be found in my book *Isometrics*, listed in the bibliography.

# MORE EXAMPLES OF APPLIED RELAXATION

Relaxation is not incompatible with safety in driving a car; on the contrary it increases efficiency and safety. Tension hastens the onset of fatigue, relaxation delays it. Tense, nervous drivers are most likely to have accidents.

The tense driver hunches forward over the steering wheel, the relaxed driver rests back against the seat. Car seats are poorly designed, so a cushion for the lower back may be necessary.

When stopped at red lights or in a traffic jam, drivers should take the opportunity to yawn and to stretch, perhaps to close the eyes briefly. These three actions are relaxing.

Drivers should let go with the muscles not needed for turning the steering wheel and working the pedals and gears. They should maintain an easy but alert sitting posture. Slumping can be as dangerous as rigidity. Relaxation is not slackness. The grip on the steering wheel should be just that needed for efficiency. Skilled drivers, including racing car drivers, learn how to economize on energy and effort.

Try differential relaxation the next time you have to sit in a dentist's chair for treatment. Instead of gazing nervously at the instruments of torture, close your eyes and let go from toes to head. Relax your face muscles, so that when the dentist asks you to open your mouth your jaw drops easily. Many people have great difficulty in lowering their jaw – it is tension and effort that keeps it up. In deep relaxation the jaw lowers spontaneously.

The examples of relaxation in activity given in this chapter are enough to indicate what is required. Once you possess the basic sense of relaxation for use in body movement – the kinaesthetic sense – it will tend to come automatically into use in whatever you do. Conscious help should be given from time to time. In this book I am concentrating on developing the basic sense of relaxation in both body and mind.

# 4 Hypnosis and Self-Hypnosis

States of deep relaxation provide an opportunity for the fruitful use of auto-suggestion. Suitably worded suggestions at such times penetrate directly to the inner mind which sets about realizing them. Advice on the most effective way to use auto-suggestion will be described in chapter 10. In the present chapter we will look at a form of deep relaxation which has the specific aim of inducing a state of heightened suggestibility.

Hypnotism had to survive many years of widespread prejudice and misunderstanding before being accepted in recent times as a valuable medical technique. The commonly used methods of induction use verbal suggestions of deep relaxation and 'sleep', and among the most significant signs of progress in deepening the hypnotic state are those indicating relaxation in the subject. That deep relaxation does occur during hypnosis is confirmed by scientific tests showing lack of tension in the skeletal muscles and the slowing down of physiological processes associated with the relaxation response investigated by Dr Herbert Benson.

The wording of the induction formula can be used to place the emphasis on releasing tension and eliciting a relaxation response. The suggestion can also be given that the subject will come out of the hypnotic state feeling refreshed and relaxed and that relaxation will permeate everyday living.

As nearly every person can learn to induce at least a light state of hypnosis in themselves, I am including an account of the method here. Hypnosis can be used for the deep relaxation it brings, and for feeding your unconscious mind suggestions for better health, recovered health, or some form of self-improvement.

## WHAT IS HYPNOSIS?

The treatment of people in trance states has been practised since ancient times, but scientists still cannot fully explain the nature of hypnosis. There is not sufficient space here to discuss the many theories put forward to explain hypnotism; not that any clear conclusion could be reached. Most general studies on hypnotism put up the theories only to show how one by one they can be toppled because they do not fit the physiological or other facts.

Brainwave patterns and other physiological responses do not fit in with the sleep theory; 'sleep' may be suggested during induction but that is to promote relaxation and not ordinary sleep. One theory held for a long time was that hypnosis was a form of hysteria and that only emotionally unstable people could be hypnotized: this has been shown to be false.

The concepts used to explain hypnosis are not themselves fully understood – suggestion, the subconscious or unconscious mind, dissociation, and so on. 'Too often in theory formation we are in the questionable position of explaining "X" by "Y" when we are not sure what "Y" is,' writes F. L. Marcuse, in *Hypnosis*, *Fact and Fiction*. He calls this 'explaining one unknown by another'.

Some investigators even take the view that 'hypnotism' does not exist, in a dispute with similarities to that over the existence or non-existence of 'dyslexia' or 'word blindness'. It is not that suggestibility does not work in dramatic ways or that some children do not have difficulty reading and writing, but whether these things can be taken out of ordinary context and given special status as it were.

'The startling truth is that there is no such thing as hypnosis,' writes Peter Blythe, in a book which he nevertheless calls *Self-Hypnosis: Its Potential and Practice*. 'The fact remains that the so-called hypnotic state does not exist when it is put under the microscope of objective investigation.'

Television performer George Kreskin has challenged anyone to produce any hypnotic phenomena that he cannot duplicate in subjects in a waking state. He has demonstrated the full range of hypnotic manifestations with wide-awake subjects. But just to further show the complexity of this inquiry, some investigators assert that responding to suggestion in the waking state is still hypnosis.

Peter Blythe says: 'Basically, waking hypnosis or the more traditional relaxing hypnosis is only an altered state of awareness allowing the uncritical acceptance of a suggestion with a concomitant involuntary response to the same suggestion.'

He also says that all people capable of adequate concentration on the instructions can be hypnotized. The 10 per cent said to be impossible to hypnotize can be hypnotized once the reason they are refusing to cooperate – 'all hypnosis is self-hypnosis' – is uncovered and removed.

Most definitions of hypnosis are based on the factor of heightened suggestibility. A fairly typical definition is that supplied by John Hartland, a medical hypnotist and psychiatrist, in *Medical and Dental Hypnosis and Its Clinical Applications*:

Hypnosis . . . is a state of mind in which suggestions are not only more readily accepted than in the waking state, but are also acted upon much more powerfully than would be possible under normal conditions. In other words, the hypnotic state is always accompanied by an increase in the suggestibility of the subject.

A definition like this still leaves us with a considerable area of mystery, but does point to the most remarkable feature of hypnosis – one that can be harnessed for useful ends.

Every day we are assaulted by suggestions, openly or insidiously – to capture our beliefs, to buy specific commercial products, and so on. It has been found that if an advertising suggestion is flashed on the television screen so rapidly that our conscious mind does not notice it, it will in fact be observed and stored in the unconscious mind. Suggestions act much more powerfully when the critical faculties of the conscious mind are bypassed and suggestions penetrate directly to the unconscious mind. This, it seems, is what happens in hypnosis. The techniques of hypnotism narrow the focus of conscious attention, promote letting go, and bring about the bypassing.

We are all familiar with being taken by surprise by some act directed by the unconscious mind when the conscious mind is preoccupied elsewhere. An example would be dialling a familiar telephone number when intending to dial another number. The hypnotic state, John Hartland says, could be looked on 'as a controlled state of absent-mindedness which can be brought on whenever one wishes, which can be terminated the moment one has no further use of it.'

Fortunately, to practise self-hypnosis and benefit from it in no way depends on siding with any particular theory about its nature, any more than our lack of knowledge about the mystery of sleep prevents us going to sleep when we retire to bed each night.

Whatever the prevailing scientific arguments, let us make use, if it suits us, of hypnotic technique in the cause of relaxed living. What concerns us is how to induce a light to medium depth hypnotic trance, how to come out of it refreshed and relaxed, and how to use hypnosis for deep relaxation, better health, and self-improvement.

## MISCONCEPTIONS

Erroneous views about hypnotism are still widespread. Probably the commonest misconception is that the subject becomes unconscious under hypnosis. Awareness continues, even in the deepest stages; the subject is aware of what is being said and what is going on.

Another misconception that can cause anxiety and resistance is that the subject is fully controlled by the hypnotist and will do anything he or she commands. However, any suggestion that goes against the moral beliefs of the subject will be resisted; if the hypnotist persists, the subject usually comes out of the trance. In self-hypnosis this particular fear need not arise.

Some people fear not being able to 'awaken' from a trance. Such problems are rare and no harm results from an extended 'sleep' anyway. In self-hypnosis the instruction can be given that you will easily terminate the session at any time you choose and for any emergency.

Another mistaken idea is that weak-willed people make the best subjects. As the subject himself or herself concentrates on the instructions and carries them out, weak-willed persons are the hardest to hypnotize because they do not concentrate sufficiently on the procedure. Conversely, strong-willed people make good subjects, provided they set their minds on being hypnotized. Being used to carrying out orders does seem to predispose people to being good subjects. For that reason, stage hypnotists will look for members of the armed forces or people in any uniform in their audiences and invite them on to the platform. Others who usually make good subjects are teenagers, nurses, actors and actresses.

The people who perform amusing antics for stage hypnotists and their audiences are usually extravert types who 'go along with' giving a performance. Thoughts about stage hypnosis need not colour one's view of the beneficial use of this therapeutic method.


## HYPNOTIC TECHNIQUE

As in other relaxation methods, you should as far as possible aim for the conditions most conducive to restfulness: a quiet room with soft lighting and freedom from avoidable distractions. The room's temperature should be neither too warm nor too cold. Wear loose-fitting clothing. The conditions, in fact, favourable to practise of progressive relaxation, and also to practise of autogenic training, biofeedback and meditation.

You should lie on your back on a firm but comfortable

surface, or sit comfortably with your feet flat on the floor and a little apart. Don't cross your legs, which impedes circulation. Rest your hands on the arms of the chair or in your lap.

The pitch of voice used in giving the instructions is important. This applies to both the voice of a hypnotist talking aloud to a subject and to your own inner voice listened to in self-hypnosis. Changes in pitch, especially when caused by excitement or by loss of confidence, could disrupt the induction process, which should proceed at an even tenor. The right tone of voice for hypnotism is calm, quiet, even and unhurried.

Relaxation is aided by closing the eyes, and in the method I am using here the eyes are closed from the start. However, quite often hypnotists ask subjects to fix their gaze on a spot on the ceiling or wall, or on a coin or other object held about two feet from the subject's face at a little above eye level. The suggestions are given that the subject is becoming sleepy, that the body is becoming heavy and that the eyes are becoming tired. These suggestions are continued for several minutes and the subject either closes his or her eyes at the suggestion 'you cannot keep your eyes open any longer' or closes them from fatigue.

There is a risk in the eye-fixation method and the suggestions, 'You cannot keep your eyes open. You want to close your eyes. Your eyes are closing. You cannot keep your eyes open any longer.' The risk is that at this early stage in the induction process the subject will say inwardly, 'Oh, yes, I can' – and keep his or her eyes open. Many hypnotists believe that this is a risk worth taking, as they can then say, in the event of failure, 'I would like you to close your eyes now. Your eyes are tired and you will relax more deeply if you close your eyes now and keep them closed.' The hypnotist hopes that this small setback will have little consequence and that the hypnotic state will come eventually. Some hypnotists take the further risk of now saying, 'Your eyes are shut fast. You are thinking of nothing but my voice. Your eyes are stuck firmly. You cannot open your eyes until I tell you to.' Failure at this point has to be met by continuing confidence in the voice and the repeated instruction that the subject will relax more deeply if he or she closes the eyes. If the eyes stay shut, the hypnotists knows the good progress is being made.

In the relaxation method that I favour, the eyes are closed from the start and tests for hypnosis need not be made until progressive relaxation is well under way through verbal suggestions. There is then no early risk of interrupting the flow of the induction procedure.

Gazing into one eye of the hypnotist is a method that is sometimes used, and it works well with some subjects, but many subjects feel uneasy at such direct contact with the hypnotist.

The connection between calm, slow breathing and relaxation is utilized in most relaxation methods, whether from East or from West. The induction suggestions include references to breathing becoming calmer, slowing down, and so on. It is helpful to say that with each exhalation tension is flowing from the body.

Suggestions of heaviness encourage letting go. Suggestions of warmth in body parts are also favourable to relaxation. These two directions are important parts of the technique of autogenic training, which is the method described in the following chapter.

The field of consciousness is narrowed and attention is kept on the instructions. If the mind wanders, it is gently brought back to the suggestions. The body stays perfectly still, the muscles 'let go' and relax. There is usually a feeling of heaviness, but some people feel a sense of lightness, perhaps of floating, and some subjects experience what seems paradoxical, heaviness and lightness. Each suggestion taken in, accepted and realized furthers progress in deepening relaxation and hypnosis.

The suggestions continue smoothly and unhurriedly for about twenty minutes. Less time is likely to be needed for induction in later sessions with the same subject.

## STAGES AND TESTS

As many as twenty different stages in the deepening of the hypnotic trance have been described in the literature of hypnosis –

but these for ordinary purposes may be reduced to three: light hypnosis, medium-depth hypnosis, and deep hypnosis or somnabulism. It is the experience of hypnotists with thousands of subjects of both sexes and all classes that 90 per cent will reach the light stage, 70 per cent the medium stage, and 20 per cent will go on to the deep stage. The deeper the hypnosis the more remarkable will be the response to suggestion. Some degree of analgesia can often be obtained in the medium-depth trance, and to a major degree in subjects in the deep trance.

Advantageous results can be obtained from suggestions given in the light stage, but medium depth is considered the best stage to induce for self-hypnotic suggestion. In the deep stage, which is harder to achieve in self-hypnosis, you are likely to lose touch with your directions.

It is probably desirable not to make any tests for hypnotic depth during the first three or four sessions. Confidence in the hypnotist and in the procedure may be marred if tests are made too soon. One should wait until there are signs of deep relaxation in the subject. The jaw muscles loosen and the lips part, while the head itself is likely to fall forward in a person sitting upright. The muscles of the face have a 'let go' look and the limbs look limp. A simple test is to tell the subject, 'I am going to lift your right hand and arm.' The arm is lifted two feet or so. 'Now I am going to let go.' If the arm is really limp it will fall like that of a rag doll.

A more advanced test, which can be tried after fifteen to twenty minutes, is to raise the dominant arm and suggest that it is becoming stiff like an iron bar. The hypnotist pulls the arm straight out from the shoulder. If the arm does become stiff, the subject is told he or she cannot bend it. If the arm cannot be bent, it is a sign of a good trance state. If the subject bends his or her arm, the hypnotist says, 'Straighten your arm. That's very good. Relax your arm now. Lower it. Fully relaxed. No longer stiff. Now go more deeply asleep. Deeper and deeper asleep,' and so on.

Another test is to suggest that the subject's right or left arm is becoming lighter and lighter and will float upwards.

Remember to return the arm to its normal weight and position.

In medium to deep states, the subject may be told that he or she will feel no pain in the hand or arm, and on being jabbed with the point of a needle will show no reaction.

Once a good trance state is established, the hypnotist or self-hypnotist can go on to give suggestions for better health or self-improvement of some kind.

## AWAKENING THE SUBJECT

Subjects are told that they will awaken easily on being told to do so, often on a count of 'one, two, three', or other sequence. They will open their eyes on 'three' and feel refreshed, alert and well.

There have been no cases of a person not awakening from hypnotic sleep, though on rare occasions a subject has had 'to sleep it off' as it were. Hypnotic trance states will turn into ordinary sleep from which the subject eventually awakens.

It is helpful to conclude hypnosis by telling subjects – or yourself in self-hypnosis – that the hypnotic state and deep relaxation will be entered quickly at the next session.

## SELF-HYPNOSIS

Most of the benefits obtained from going to a professional hypnotist may be obtained through self-hypnosis. Light to medium trance states are easily achieved by most people and provide a hypersuggestible state that can be utilized as you wish for repeating self-improvement phrases worded to meet your specific needs, or for its enjoyable deep relaxation and replenishment of physical and mental energies. Even deep-rooted stresses may be released.

Self-hypnosis is safe. But one precaution should be observed – to always remove any suggestion or phenomena before awakening.

The verbal suggestions of the induction formula are set out in a form for easy purusal, memorization or tape recording.

You can make your own recording or have a friend do it, changing the wording from the first person into the third person.

Commercial tape recordings for inducing hypnosis often fail for a variety of reasons. They are fixed and cannot adapt to individual needs; the subject may not like the sound of the recorded voice or the stranger's voice may arouse the conscious censor who says, 'No, I will not cooperate'; if they have a musical background, it will not be to every subject's taste (it is often a mushy strings sound); the wording cannot be changed.

Your own tape recording is a better idea, for you can be certain it meets your needs. If you do not like the sound of your own voice, you can ask a friend to make the recording; but any unfamiliar intonation or uneven rhythm in the voice may cause mild but persistent irritation.

The best method of self-hypnosis is to learn the formula and stay in full control without reliance on artificial aids. If you can become word perfect – fine! But it is necessary only to keep the suggestions moving slowly and smoothly on the general lines, with your own slight adaptations of the wording if you wish, of deepening relaxation and deepening hypnotic sleep. Suggestions of letting go, of heaviness, of release of tension, of limpness, of breathing deeply and calmly, of feeling peaceful, and so on. Keep on repeating the suggestions in an even, quiet, soothing tone.

The induction formula is voiced inwardly in self-hypnosis and listened to, while sitting comfortably or lying on your back, in a quiet, softly lit room in which there are few distractions.

## INDUCTION FORMULA FOR SELF-HYPNOSIS

I settle comfortably in the chair. Or: I lie on my back relaxed
   and comfortable
I close my eyes
I listen to my inner voice
I concentrate fully on what I am saying
I think of nothing else

I am going to relax deeply
I am going to relax completely
I am going to sink into hypnotic sleep
I am going to enjoy refreshing relaxation and hypnotic sleep
I am thinking of nothing but what I tell myself
I go along with what is happening
I go along with the drift into deep relaxation
Already I am becoming more relaxed and comfortable
I go along with what is happening
I go along with the drift into deep relaxation
I am letting go and sinking into relaxation
I am letting go and sinking into deeper relaxation
I am letting it happen as it happens
No problems trouble me
I let it happen
Nothing matters but drifting into pleasant relaxation
I let deep relaxation come
I let deep sleep come
I am paying full attention to this formula
I am listening to my words and not thinking of anything else
Soon I will be deeply relaxed and in hypnotic sleep
I will awaken easily when I want to or for an emergency
I will awaken feeling refreshed and relaxed
I will awaken feeling peaceful and well
I am letting go and sinking into deeper relaxation
I am letting go and sinking into deeper relaxation
I am aware of my breathing
I am aware of my breathing
I take a slow, deep breath
I let the breath out slowly
I think of tension flowing out of my body
I take another slow, deep breath
I let the breath out slowly
I think of tension flowing out of my body
I breathe deep in my abdomen
I breathe deep in my abdomen
I feel my abdomen rise and fall, calmly and gently

I feel my abdomen rise and fall, calmly and gently
I let my breathing happen
My breathing is slow
My breathing is slow
My breathing is deep
My breathing is deep
My breathing is calm
My breathing is calm
My breathing is slow, deep and calm
My breathing is slow, deep and calm
With each breathing out I become more calm and deeply
   relaxed
With each breathing out I become more deeply relaxed
With each breathing out I become more deeply asleep
With each breathing out I become more deeply asleep
I am breathing freely
I am breathing freely
I am enjoying calm, relaxed breathing
I am enjoying calm, relaxed breathing
With each letting out of breath I drift deeper into relaxation
With each letting out of breath I drift deeper into relaxation
With each letting out of breath I drift deeper into sleep
With each letting out of breath I drift deeper into sleep
I find myself relaxing more and more with each breath I take
I find myself relaxing more and more with each breath I take
Nothing matters but letting go
Nothing matters but relaxing more deeply
From toes to scalp, I am relaxing more deeply
From toes to scalp, I am relaxing more deeply
I am relaxing completely
All tensions going
Every drop of tension going
I let go with all my muscles
I let go with all my muscles
I allow all my muscles to go limp
I allow all my muscles to go limp
From toes to scalp, my muscles feel relaxed and limp

From toes to scalp, my muscles feel relaxed and limp
My right foot feels limp and relaxed
My right foot feels limp and relaxed
My right lower leg feels limp and relaxed
My right lower leg feels limp and relaxed
My right knee feels limp and relaxed
My right knee feels limp and relaxed
My right upper leg feels limp and relaxed
My right upper leg feels limp and relaxed
My right buttock and hip feel limp and relaxed
My right buttock and hip feel limp and relaxed
My right leg from foot to hip feels limp and relaxed
My right leg from foot to hip feels limp and relaxed
My left foot feels limp and relaxed
My left foot feels limp and relaxed
My left lower leg feels limp and relaxed
My left lower leg feels limp and relaxed
My left knee feels limp and relaxed
My left knee feels limp and relaxed
My left upper leg feels limp and relaxed
My left upper leg feels limp and relaxed
My left buttock and hip feels limp and relaxed
My left buttock and hip feels limp and relaxed
My left leg from foot to hip feels limp and relaxed
My left leg from foot to hip feels limp and relaxed
My lower abdomen feels limp and relaxed
My lower abdomen feels limp and relaxed
My upper abdomen feels limp and relaxed
My upper abdomen feels limp and relaxed
My lower back feels limp and relaxed
My lower back feels limp and relaxed
My upper back feels limp and relaxed
My upper back feels limp and relaxed
My chest muscles feel limp and relaxed
My chest muscles feel limp and relaxed
I breathe freely
I breathe freely

My breathing is free and deep
My breathing is free and deep
My legs and torso feel limp and relaxed
My right hand feels limp and relaxed
My right hand feels limp and relaxed
My right forearm feels limp and relaxed
My right forearm feels limp and relaxed
My right elbow feels limp and relaxed
My right elbow feels limp and relaxed
My right upper arm feels limp and relaxed
My right upper arm feels limp and relaxed
My right shoulder feels limp and relaxed
My right shoulder feels limp and relaxed
My right arm from hand to shoulder feels limp and relaxed
My right arm from hand to shoulder feels limp and relaxed
I breathe freely and deeply
I breathe freely and deeply
My left hand feels limp and relaxed
My left hand feels limp and relaxed
My left forearm feels limp and relaxed
My left forearm feels limp and relaxed
My left elbow feels limp and relaxed
My left elbow feels limp and relaxed
My left upper arm feels limp and relaxed
My left upper arm feels limp and relaxed
My left shoulder feels limp and relaxed
My left shoulder feels limp and relaxed
My left arm from hand to shoulder feels limp and relaxed
My left arm from hand to shoulder feels limp and relaxed
I breathe freely and deeply
I breathe freely and deeply
My neck feels limp and relaxed
My neck feels limp and relaxed
My jaws feel limp and relaxed
My jaws feel limp and relaxed
My mouth feels limp and relaxed
My mouth feels limp and relaxed

My cheeks feel limp and relaxed
My cheeks feel limp and relaxed
My eyelids feel limp and relaxed
My eyelids feel limp and relaxed
My forehead feels limp and relaxed
My forehead feels limp and relaxed
My scalp feels limp and relaxed
My scalp feels limp and relaxed
From feet to head, I feel limp and relaxed
From feet to head, I feel limp and relaxed
My eyes are closed and I do not want to open them
My eyes are closed and I do not want to open them
I breathe freely
I breathe freely
With every breath I take I become more and more deeply
     relaxed
With every breath I take I become more and more deeply
     relaxed
I feel pleasantly heavy and drowsy
I feel pleasantly heavy and drowsy
I am relaxing completely
I am relaxing completely
From feet to scalp, I am letting go
From feet to scalp, I am letting go
My whole body feels heavy and relaxed
My whole body feels heavy and relaxed
From feet to scalp, I feel heavy and relaxed
From feet to scalp, I feel heavy and relaxed
My right foot feels heavy and relaxed
My right foot feels heavy and relaxed
My right lower leg feels heavy and relaxed
My right lower leg feels heavy and relaxed
My right knee feels heavy and relaxed
My right knee feels heavy and relaxed
My right upper leg feels heavy and relaxed
My right upper leg feels heavy and relaxed
My right buttock and hip feel heavy and relaxed

My right buttock and hip feel heavy and relaxed
My right leg feels heavy and relaxed
My right leg feels heavy and relaxed
My left foot feels heavy and relaxed
My left foot feels heavy and relaxed
My left lower leg feels heavy and relaxed
My left lower leg feels heavy and relaxed
My left knee feels heavy and relaxed
My left knee feels heavy and relaxed
My left upper leg feels heavy and relaxed
My left upper leg feels heavy and relaxed
My left buttock and hip feel heavy and relaxed
My left buttock and hip feel heavy and relaxed
My left leg from foot to hip feels heavy and relaxed
My left leg from foot to hip feels heavy and relaxed
My lower abdomen feels heavy and relaxed
My lower abdomen feels heavy and relaxed
My upper abdomen feels heavy and relaxed
My upper abdomen feels heavy and relaxed
My lower back feels heavy and relaxed
My lower back feels heavy and relaxed
My breathing is free and deep
My breathing is free and deep
My upper back feels heavy and relaxed
My upper back feels heavy and relaxed
My breathing is free and deep
My breathing is free and deep
My legs and torso feel heavy and relaxed
My right hand feels heavy and relaxed
My right hand feels heavy and relaxed
My right forearm feels heavy and relaxed
My right forearm feels heavy and relaxed
My right elbow feels heavy and relaxed
My right elbow feels heavy and relaxed
My right upper arm feels heavy and relaxed
My right upper arm feels heavy and relaxed
My right shoulder feels heavy and relaxed

My right shoulder feels heavy and relaxed
My right arm from hand to shoulder feels heavy and relaxed
My right arm from hand to shoulder feels heavy and relaxed
I breathe freely and deeply
I breathe freely and deeply
My left hand feels heavy and relaxed
My left hand feels heavy and relaxed
My left forearm feels heavy and relaxed
My left forearm feels heavy and relaxed
My left elbow feels heavy and relaxed
My left elbow feels heavy and relaxed
My left upper arm feels heavy and relaxed
My left upper arm feels heavy and relaxed
My left shoulder feels heavy and relaxed
My left shoulder feels heavy and relaxed
My left arm from hand to shoulder feels heavy and relaxed
My left arm from hand to shoulder feels heavy and relaxed
I breathe freely and deeply
I breathe freely and deeply
I feel comfortable and peaceful
I feel comfortable and peaceful
My neck feels heavy and relaxed
My neck feels heavy and relaxed
My jaws feel heavy and relaxed
My jaws feel heavy and relaxed
My eyelids feel heavy and relaxed
My eyelids feel heavy and relaxed
My forehead feels heavy and relaxed
My forehead feels heavy and relaxed
My head feels heavy and relaxed
My head feels heavy and relaxed
My legs, torso, arms, and head feel heavy and relaxed
My legs, torso, arms, and head feel heavy and relaxed
My whole body feels deeply relaxed
My whole body feels deeply relaxed
I feel pleasantly heavy and drowsy
I feel pleasantly heavy and drowsy

I am drifting into hypnotic sleep
I am drifting into hypnotic sleep
I am drifting further and further into hypnotic sleep
I am drifting further and further into hypnotic sleep
I let go to hypnotic sleep
I let go to hypnotic sleep
I give myself up completely to relaxing sleep
I give myself up completely to relaxing sleep
I am going sound asleep
I am going sound asleep
Nothing matters except going sound asleep
Nothing matters except going sound asleep
I am sinking into deep, sound sleep
I am sinking into deep, sound sleep
As I count slowly inwardly from one to ten, I will feel more and
   more relaxed and deeper and deeper asleep
As I count slowly inwardly from one to ten, I will feel more and
   more relaxed and deeper and deeper asleep
One . . . two . . . three . . . more and more relaxed
Four . . . five . . . six . . . deeper and deeper asleep
Seven . . . eight . . . nine . . . more and more relaxed and
   deeper and deeper asleep
Ten . . . deeply asleep
Deeply asleep
Deeply asleep
Deeply asleep
As I count slowly inwardly from one to ten, I will feel more and
   more relaxed and deeper and deeper asleep
As I count slowly inwardly from one to ten, I will feel more and
   more relaxed and deeper and deeper asleep
One . . . two . . . three . . . more and more relaxed
Four . . . five . . . six . . . deeper and deeper asleep
Seven . . . eight . . . nine . . . more and more relaxed and
   deeper and deeper asleep
Ten . . . deeply asleep
Deeply asleep
Deeply asleep
Deeply asleep

Enjoy the self-hypnotic relaxation for as many minutes more as you wish. Before coming out of hypnosis, you may wish at this point to take full advantage of the state to give some realistic positive suggestions of recovering health if needed, of improved health, of greater calmness and confidence in living, of not smoking or overeating or some other habit you would like to break, and so on. This is also the time to test the depth of your state of hypnosis, if you wish, though this should not be done until you have had at least four or five sessions of self-hypnosis. Make sure you remove any suggestions or phenomena before awakening.

## RIGIDITY TEST

I am lifting my right arm (or left arm, according to which is
    dominant) straight out from my shoulder
My arm is straight out and becoming very stiff
My arm is becoming stiffer and stiffer
Now my raised arm is as rigid as an iron bar
I cannot bend my arm
It will not bend
I try to bend my raised arm
The arm is rigid and will not bend
It is like an iron bar
I try to bend it again
It will not bend
Now I relax my raised right (or left) arm
The rigidity is draining away
My right (or left) arm is no longer stiff
My right (or left) arm is normal now and I can bend it
My raised arm is normal and I lower my arm to its resting
    position
Both my arms are relaxed
Now I go more deeply asleep
I am relaxed and deeply asleep

# WEIGHTLESS TEST

Suggest your dominant arm is becoming weightless and floating upwards.

My right (or left) arm is becoming lighter and lighter
Its weight is dissolving
All weight is going out of the arm
My right (or left) arm is becoming light as a feather
My arm is becoming lighter and lighter
Soon my right (or left) arm will start bending and floating
  upwards
Lighter and lighter, lighter and lighter
No weight in the arm
My right (or left) arm is bending and starting to rise
Hand and arm starting to float upwards
Bending and floating upwards

Bend and raise the arm slightly if it hasn't risen involuntarily.

My weightless right (or left) arm is floating upwards
Soon my hand will float up and touch my face
My hand is floating up slowly towards my face
Soon it will touch my face
My weightless arm is floating up
Hand coming up to face

Whether your hand has touched your face or not, say:

Now my right (or left) arm is returning to its normal weight
Normal weight is back in the arm
I lower the arm to its former position
My right (or left) arm has returned to its normal weight and
  resting position

# AWAKENING

In a few moments, in the time it takes me to count from five
  back to zero, I will open my eyes and awaken from hypnotic
  sleep
All tiredness and heaviness will have gone

I will feel alert, relaxed and refreshed

This feeling will stay with me as I go about my day-to-day activities

Next time I practise self-hypnosis, I will sink rapidly into pleasant, relaxing hypnotic sleep. I will quickly become deeply relaxed and deeply asleep

But now, as I count backwards from five to zero, I will awaken, feeling alert and peaceful

Five . . . Four . . . beginning to awaken

Three . . . Two . . . awakening, awakening

One . . . nearly awake

Zero . . . eyes open and awake

## RAPID INDUCTION

Once you are experienced with the full induction formula, often a few key phrases may be used to trigger quick hypnotic relaxation. This is useful for taking five minutes' or so rest when fatigued, or before going out in the evening. It is particularly useful at times of crisis or just before an important event, especially one in which you are likely to feel nervous. At such times, while in deep relaxation, you should suggest to yourself that you will cope with the important event calmly and effectively, giving it your full concentration.

Select a few key phrases, such as 'letting go', 'heavy and relaxed all over', and 'deeply relaxed'. In time, the two words 'deeply relaxed', spoken inwardly with emphasis may be enough to trigger instant relaxation.

For rapid induction, the one to ten count that is used twice in the preceding induction formula may be adapted.

One . . . two . . . three . . . letting go

Four . . . five . . . six . . . breathing slow, deep, and calm.

Seven . . . body heavy and relaxed

Eight . . . heavy and relaxed all over

Nine . . . deeper and deeper relaxed

Ten . . . deeply relaxed (with emphasis)

## USES OF HYPNOSIS

In this chapter hypnosis has been described as a relaxation method. Deep relaxation is characteristic of the state of hypnosis, but the value of this component has tended to be overshadowed by a more sensational element – hypersuggesti-bility. This results from the way the induction techniques lull the conscious mind – at any rate that part of it which acts as the censor and filter of incoming suggestions – into a quiescent state, so that suggestions, whether negative or positive, pene-trate straight into the subconscious or unconscious mind and are acted upon automatically. Hypnotherapy and the use of hypnosis for self-improvement makes use of the potency of positive suggestions agreed in advance with a hypnotist or given by yourself in self-hypnosis.

Discussion of these uses of auto-suggestion and hypnosis has been reserved for a later chapter, because auto-suggestion func-tions well in states of deep relaxation and passivity, whether they are achieved by hypnosis or by any of the other methods described in this book.

The lighter states of hypnotic trance are often indistin-guishable from the subjective experience of the consciousness associated with other forms of deep relaxation. Even objective scientific investigators have difficulty in agreeing on the nature of distinctions between altered states of consciousness.

Even if you are not a person who slips easily into the hypnotic state, using the preceding self-hypnosis induction formula will, if faithfully followed, produce a worthwhile relaxation experi-ence. But if you feel that self-hypnosis, for one reason or another, is not for you, or has no special advantages over other methods, there remain the techniques of progressive relaxation, biofeedback, meditation, and one that developed out of a psychiatrist's desire that the therapeutic benefits of hypnosis should be available to all patients, and which may or may not be a form itself of self-hypnosis. This method is the subject of our next chapter.

# 5 Autogenic Training

## WHAT IS AUTOGENIC TRAINING?

Autogenic training is a therapy devised by a German psychiatrist, Johannes H. Schultz, in the 1920s. He called it *autogene training*. Training is the same word in German and in English and autogene or autogenic comes from combining two Greek words – *auto*, meaning 'self', and *genous*, meaning 'originated'. Schultz wrote a book on his therapy – sometimes called autogenics – which was published in Stuttgart in 1932 and which has been reprinted many times. Many hundreds of medical papers have been written about autogenic training. The main centres of practice have been in continental Europe, particularly in Germany and Switzerland; its use in Britain and in the United States of America has been much less, but is now growing rapidly.

Autogenics is a mixture of auto-suggestion, self-hypnosis, Yoga-like conscious control over physiologic functions normally regulated by the autonomic nervous system, exercise of the imagination, and meditation. The meaning of the word 'autogenic' points to its being a self-help relaxation therapy. The individual lies down, or sometimes sits, relaxes and responds to a series of auto-suggestions, whose order and phrasing are important. Teachers of the method consider that each subject should be instructed in the training programme before operating it himself or herself at home. However, a great many people have learned the technique from books. Success will come more easily if you are already familiar with one or more of such awareness practices as progressive relaxation, biofeedback or meditation. Poised attention is the key to success in autogenic training as it is in the other deep relaxation methods.

In autogenic training, as in self-hypnosis, you direct attention away from the external environment and focus on body sensations of heaviness and warmth – conditions favourable to both muscular and vascular relaxation, to self-healing, and to opening the subconscious for the implanting of beneficial seed suggestions.

Johannes Schultz read all he could about Yoga and other Eastern psychophysical disciplines – his therapy is sometimes called a kind of Western Yoga. He also studied and used hypnosis and auto-suggestion. Only a few years before, Emile Coué had propagated his auto-suggestion therapy, with its popularized basic therapeutic sentence: 'Every day in every way, I am getting better and better.' Schultz saw that in a state of deep relaxation combined with passive awareness it was possible to become aware of body sensations normally overlaid by external sensory impressions or the mind's thought-chatter. Similar awareness of our internal environment occurs during meditation, in which there is sense withdrawal and quietening of the mind.

The next step for Schultz was Yogic-like control of some physiological functions normally regulated only by the autonomic (involuntary) nervous system: by passive awareness and repeating phrases of an auto-suggestive or self-hypnotic type – 'my heartbeat is calm and strong', 'my right hand is getting warm', 'my solar plexus feels warm and glowing'. Some beginners can achieve a rise in hand temperature of 2° Fahrenheit, and with practice rises of up to 10° are recorded. You can put in some preliminary practice now by strapping a household thermometer to one hand and thinking of warmth in the whole hand. In a few minutes the mercury should start to rise and acts as a biofeedback signal that aids progress. If you don't succeed immediately, try again later, always staying relaxed and not forcing a result.

It is important that the subjective experience of autogenic

training should be remembered and carried as far as possible into everyday living. Autogenics embraces a broader spectrum of goals than releasing nervous tension, relieving pain and treating illness. Its highest goal is the cultivation of a special quality of living, which in this book I have called poised living. Progressive relaxation, auto-suggestion, self-hypnosis, biofeedback and meditation can also be used with this purpose in mind.

Dr Karl Robert Rosa, in his book *Autogenic Training*, defines the system as 'the art of self-discovery and the means to a new, relaxed enjoyment of one's pure existence', which I could say are two of the principal aims of this book. In advanced stages, autogenics employs the imaginative powers of the mind and meditative techniques that some operators take to mystical or near mystical reaches, though Schultz himself did not describe his goals in religious terms. His book *Das Autogene Training* bore the subtitle 'Concentrated Self-Relaxation', which is what we focus on in this chapter; but he was aware that deep relaxation is linked not only to good health of body and mind but also to values and attitudes, psychic freedom and breadth of experience.

Dr Wolfgang Kretschmer Jr, of the Tübingen University Psychiatric Clinic, wrote an article for a German medical magazine on 'Meditative Techniques in Psychotherapy', in which he said that Schultz

limits himself to the formulation of basic existential values. This means the meditator is encouraged to strive toward a reasonable view of life oriented toward self-realization, psychic freedom and harmony, and a lively creativity. At best, one achieves a Nirvana-like phenomenon of joy and release. Maybe Schultz conceals decisive experiences which go further; because of the basically unlimited possibilities of meditation, we can always await such an extension of his ideas.

## AUTOGENICS AND HYPNOSIS

In 1929 Johannes Schultz said: 'Autogenic training was developed in direct connection with my experiences with hypnosis.' He had used hypnosis with his patients, but sought a method of treatment that was free from certain of hypnosis's drawbacks – particularly the fundamental problems that not all patients could be hypnotized and that results for the others were often erratic.

Some subjects resist coming under the control of the hypnotist. In autogenic training the patient is in control and follows his or her own suggestions. Nevertheless, the state of consciousness induced by autogenic training is often described as 'light hypnosis', 'shallow hypnosis', 'a light hypnoid state', and so on. Verbal suggestions of the kind described earlier are used for inducing self-hypnosis. Self-hypnosis? The hypnagogic state (bordering on sleep)? Deep relaxation through auto-suggestion? Meditative consciousness? States of consciousness are still mysterious seas in process of scientific charting.

If a relaxation method works, we need not worry too much about the labels attached. If you feel uncomfortable about the idea of even light self-directed hypnotic trance, I would advise you to try the programme and judge your comfort or discomfort with it for yourself. Few people find the experience other than deeply pleasurable.

## THE AUTOGENIC STATE

The state attained in autogenic training should not be confused with listlessness, drowsiness or ordinary sleep. The conscious mind becomes very quiet; there is passive awareness and effortless concentration on the body and some of its physiological processes. There is deep relaxation of the skeletal muscles, which, if evidence of studies in progressive relaxation apply here, also extends to smooth muscle. The opposing paired muscles (the antagonists) settle down to take a well-earned rest from their alternating contractions and expansions. There is a reduction of the state of muscle tone by which the body keeps ready for action and its functions active.

The blood vessels are dilated; this is especially so in the extremities, so that there is a more even distribution of blood throughout the body. This is experienced as a feeling of warmth suffusing the body. In addition, there is heightened warmth in the hands and the solar plexus, on which awareness dwells. Heartbeat slows down slightly and respiration and oxygen consumption considerably. Dr Karl Rosa uses the term 'vegetative relaxation' for the way in which the abdominal area is suffused with warmth and the abdominal organs function smoothly.

In contrast to the hands, the abdomen, and the rest of the body, the head feels cool – 'a cool, de-concentrated head' Schultz called it. In other words, the body is deeply relaxed but the attention stays alert, poised and watchful. Thoughts move quietly and slowly through the mind and are reduced in number: gaps between thoughts are experienced and observed lucid and pure. There is a calm choiceless awareness in the manner of most Eastern meditation. Awareness is limited to body sensations. There is a sense of warm relaxation and of passive pleasure. 'The return', as it is called – coming back to everyday active living – is characterized by replenished energies, a sense of wellbeing, calmness and clarity of mind.

In short, autogenic training induces the relaxation response described in chapter 1 – the opposite of the fight-or-flight response to danger in which the body mobilizes for great effort. And the relaxation response promotes healing and freedom from fear and anxiety.

## THE AUTOGENIC FORMULAE

Advanced stages of autogenics may bring in fantasy and quasi-mystical elements, Dr Roberto Assaglio pointed out in his *Psychosynthesis*, that 'unfortunately' these 'higher stages' have been written about 'only in the vaguest form'. But what concerns us here is the basic deep relaxation programme, described by Dr Karl Rosa as 'a complete and independent practicable method'. Its six parts are usually described as 'standard exercises', but Schultz liked to call them *einstellungen* – 'orientations'. Each part is based on a verbal formula seeking to influence some part of the body. There is no doubt that the basic autogenic programme is an effective method of self-inducing psychophysical relaxation that is subjectively experienced as integrating and harmonious for body and mind.

The six 'orientations' in sequence are as follows:

1. *Right arm (left, if left-handed) becoming heavy.* A sense of heaviness, of letting go with the arm, supported perhaps by imagining it to be made of lead or some other weighty matter, leads to relaxation in the arm and to sympathetic relaxation elsewhere in the body.

2. *Right hand (left, if left-handed) becoming warm.* The suggestion is repeated several times and awareness is focused steadily but without strain on the hand until it becomes warm. Preliminary practice on the lines suggested earlier (strapping a household thermometer to the hand), is helpful. If warmth does not increase noticeably after five minutes of directed attention to the hand, move on to stage 3 and return after completing the programme to stage 2. It makes the exercise easier if you imagine the hand is in a patch of strong sunlight, or receiving the warmth of a fire. Otherwise all you have to do is let the attention dwell on the hand steadily and repeat the suggestion of its being suffused with warmth.

3. *Pulse calm and strong.* The heartbeat can be reduced by several beats per minute through this verbal suggestion. A slower pulse rate is an indication of greater calmness and relaxation, and the heart continues to function efficiently. A minority of people become anxious at any thought of the heart. The relaxation programme should itself remove or reduce that fear. If it persists strongly in early practice, it would be best for that person to eliminate the third formula from training until such time as it can be included without producing any tension. Some people may find the suggestion 'strong' too indicative of action; for them 'pulse calm' would suffice as a formula.

4. *Breathing calm and regular.* Here we have the age-old wisdom of the East. Quiet, even breathing (poised breathing) is essential for the ancient and modern practice of meditation: the relaxing effect is obvious. When a person is anxious, fearful or agitated,

respiration becomes rapid, uneven and shallow; when a person is calm and composed, breathing is slow, regular and deep into the abdomen. Note that your breathing will naturally become slower as relaxation deepens. You should not interfere with the flow of breath apart from repeating the formula. The suggestion 'Breathing calm and regular' is allowed to do its work through passive awareness: this is not a breathing 'exercise' of the kind that is part of the Hatha Yoga (physical yoga) system. Some manuals on autogenics include the formula 'It breathes me' at this stage. This is in line with Eastern techniques of meditation based on awareness of breathing. The big metaphysical question is: what is the 'it' that breathes you?

5. *Solar plexus warm*. This formula also has affinities with Oriental spiritual and psychophysical training. As discussed elsewhere in this book, Japanese mysticism, culture and sport attach great importance to the *tanden* or 'vital belly centre' and to *hara* which is a concept embracing the whole abdominal area and the centre of gravity of the body. The tanden is about two fingers' width below the navel and the solar plexus about the same distance above it. The solar plexus is a very important centre for the nervous system. The name 'solar' is fortunate, with its suggestion of glowing heat. The whole abdomen becomes suffused with warmth, encouraging muscular and vascular relaxation. It helps to have an image of a fiery sun in the area: warmth is healing. Learning to create sensations of warmth in any body part through directed awareness is a valuable skill to cultivate. It can be used at times when the body is uncomfortably cold or when a body part is unhealthy or damaged and would benefit from warmth. Such localized awareness can also relieve and remove pain.

6. *Forehead pleasantly cool*. The head is the only part of the body to become cool; the arms, trunk, and legs will become more relaxed if they are warm. The helpful image here can be of body in sunshine but head in shade. Schultz instructed his patients to visualize a mountain with subtropical vegetation around its base but its peak snow-capped. Note that the head should feel

pleasantly cool – not cold! This is an important distinction. A cool head and warm feet for good health is part of the folk medicine of several countries. A German proverb says: 'Cool head, warm feet – that makes the best doctor poor!'

Note, too, that a cool head represents poised attention, not thinking. Consciousness stays calm and alertly poised during autogenic training. It is true that if you are very tired you may become drowsy or pass into sleep. If you do take a nap, complete the programme on waking.

Terminating the autogenic training programme is not a problem. You are in control throughout and need do no more than make a decision to end the programme with a slow count from five back to zero. Then sit up and wait a minute or so before standing up. On resuming everyday activities try to carry the feeling of deep relaxation with you. For several hours the relaxation response will stay with you as an 'afterglow'.

Schultz called the termination of the programme *Zurücknahme* – 'return'. The method he favoured now seems unnecessarily vigorous. He instructed: (1) arms firm, flexing them strongly like a comic-strip strongman; (2) deep breath; (3) eyes open.

I prefer to stretch the legs on a count of 'five'; stretch the arms on a count of 'four'; stretch the arms and legs on a count of 'three'; take a deep breath and let it out like a sigh on a count of 'two'; open the eyes on a count of 'one'; sit up slowly, yawning and stretching, at 'zero'. This gives a smooth transition to the active state.

The formulas' phrases should be brief and sum up an 'orientation' whose image is clear and can be converted into awareness. They can be supported by any visualizations that help produce the intended effect, such as a solid weight for the arms, sunlight and shade, or a snow-capped mountain. If any words strike a wrong note with you – giving rise to thoughts that might cause disharmony rather than harmony, tension rather than relaxation – latitude is allowed in the wording of the formulas as long as the basic structure is followed.

After a few months, when you have become expert in

autogenic training, you will find that the formulas can be shortened to just a word or two at each stage. These will be enough to trigger the response. Here are examples: (1) 'arm' or 'heaviness'; (2) 'hand' or 'warmth'; (3) 'pulse' or 'calm'; (4) 'breathing', 'calm' or 'regular'; (5) 'solar', 'plexus' or 'warm'; (6) 'cool' or 'forehead'.

The style and tone of voice used in giving the verbal suggestions to yourself, to another person, or recording them on tape should be as advised for hypnosis and self-hypnosis. The voice should be quiet but firm, unhurried, soothing, calm and steady. If in making a recording you falter at some point in a way that could prove irritating in listening to the tape, remake that section. If you hate your own voice, have some other person make the recording for you.

Poised attention, relaxed yet alert, is the key to success in autogenics, just as in meditation. There is concentration, but effortless concentration which is the key factor in Oriental meditation and Zen art and sport . . . indeed, Zen living. Dr Rosa says: 'The subject, in the autogenic training state, is aware of himself in all his senses but does not reflect on himself', and he calls this 'a pleasant state of being'. The same words could be used of the meditative state. Focus is achieved without thought other than that suggested by the formula. Each time you find your attention has wavered, bring it gently back to the formula. Leave gaps of silence between verbal suggestions in which they take effect, but not so long that distracting thoughts occur. Keep to the suggestions without adding thoughts. Your attitude should be one of non-striving and non-grasping. Passively wait for relaxation and warmth to come. 'Over and above all else the trainee must be willing to let it happen,' says Dr Rosa.

Some explanation is required for the programme which I have set out line by line below, in a manner similar to that given earlier for self-hypnosis, to facilitate memorization or recording.

It has become commonplace in using autogenics in Britain and in the United States of America to combine it with some elements of progressive relaxation, extending the range of directed awareness to both arms (not just the dominant arm), to the facial muscles, the shoulders, the back, the hips, and the legs and feet, while retaining the verbal suggestion method of autogenics. I follow that course below, for which recent scientific research gives some justification. Some investigators have found that relaxing one body part – say a hand – does not necessarily relax the whole body, though some parts relax sympathetically. The more skilled you are in relaxation the more likely it becomes that general relaxation follows letting go from tension in selected parts. If you become very skilled in the neuromuscular art you may be able to achieve a high degree of overall psychophysical relaxation through relaxing just one hand or arm – but that is unlikely for beginners, and by no means certain even for experienced trainees.

So I have given greater overall coverage in relaxation in the programme given below, in which all main muscle groups receive the tension-dissolving touch of poised awareness. Some elements of proved value from the techniques of self-hypnosis are also incorporated – repetition of key phrases, for example. These combinations are justified by their effectiveness. Later, as mentioned a few paragraphs earlier, you will find that the whole programme can be concentrated in a few key words to which you have been conditioned to respond, bringing warmth and deep relaxation to the body and a soothing coolness to the head.

## PREPARATIONS

Occasionally, autogenic training may be practised sitting in a chair, but the usual position for going through the standard exercises is as already described for the practice of progressive relaxation. Lie supine on a couch, firm bed or on the floor with a carpet, rug or folded blanket beneath you to prevent discomfort. Your head, trunk, arms and legs should be distributed symmetrically. Your head should be in line with your spine and you look straight upwards. Spread your back and keep every part of it in contact with the surface you are lying on. The lower back, too, should make contact, though some people will not manage this fully until after they have had some postural training; following the advice given in chapter 2 will help with this. Your arms should lie limply alongside your torso and a little apart from it, your hands unclenched and fingers loose. Your feet should be slightly apart and your toes falling outwards. Let go with your whole body so that you feel you are lying with your full weight; there should be no feelings of rigidity. Some people may wish to place small cushions behind the neck and under the lower back.

Wear loose-fitting clothing and remove or loosen any constricting garments: take off your shoes and stockings. Wash at least your face and hands shortly before practice, and visit the toilet. Blow each nostril separately into your handkerchief, and waggle a finger gently in each ear for a few seconds.

The room in which you practice should be the quietest available, softly lighted, of comfortable temperature, the air pleasantly fresh and draught-free. If you are likely to feel cold, cover yourself with a blanket. Distractions of all kinds should be kept to a minimum. *Do not disturb* is the message.

Practise twice a day, each session lasting ten to thirty minutes – twenty minutes is a good period to settle on. Or once a day with progressive relaxation, self-hypnosis, or meditation occupying the other session.

A final reminder about attitude. For autogenics we need 'a passive casual attitude'. You are going to relax, not strive to perform amazing feats. Remember what Schultz said: 'The system works automatically, you do not do it.'

This impersonal, egoless attitude, which is akin to that of meditation, is aided by dropping references to 'I' and 'my' in the verbal suggestions. This does not matter to any real extent in self-hypnosis, and phrasing of the 'I' and 'my' type are given in many accounts of autogenic training – but this seems to me a wrong approach. I prefer 'forehead pleasantly cool' to 'my forehead is pleasantly cool'. I am not saying that success cannot be achieved using 'I' and 'my' phrases and it is difficult to avoid their use if you choose to make use of autogenic relaxation for auto-suggestion aiming at self-improvement of some kind. But I believe the more impersonal formula elicits the right effortless attitude: poised awareness can be trusted to carry on its beneficial work.

The programme opens with a condensed tense and 'let go' procedure which, especially if you are already advancing with training in progressive relaxation, will give a good start for head to toe relaxation.

## AUTOGENIC RELAXATION PROGRAMME

Resting comfortably, eyes closed
Breathing easily
Taking slow, deep breaths
Lying with your full weight
Letting go and settling down
Breathing slowly and deeply
Letting tension go
Pulling toes and instep towards face, contracting right leg strongly from foot to hip
Letting go from contraction of right leg
Right leg limp and relaxed
Taking easy, deep breaths
Deep easy breathing
Pulling toes and instep towards face, contracting left leg strongly from foot to hip
Letting go from contraction of left leg
Left leg limp and relaxed
Breathing slowly and deeply
Making a fist with right hand and squeezing tightly, tightening whole arm strongly from hand to shoulder
Letting go from contraction, relaxing the arm
Right arm limp and relaxed
Taking slow, deep breaths
Making a fist of the left hand and squeezing tightly, tightening whole arm strongly from hand to shoulder
Letting go from contraction, relaxing the arm
Left arm limp and relaxed
Both arms limp and relaxed from hands to shoulders
Breathing slowly and deeply

Tightening tummy muscles and pressing down with back and head

Letting go from tension in abdomen and upper body

Tension flowing away

Breathing slowly and deeply

Bringing lips together and pressing them together firmly, contracting facial muscles from chin to scalp

Face relaxing and broadening, thinking of smiling

Taking a slow, deep breath

Holding breath and contracting all body muscles from feet to scalp

Letting breath out through mouth, relaxing whole body

Tension flowing out and whole body relaxed and comfortable

Letting go from tension with every breathing out

Breathing calm and regular

Lying with full weight and letting go

Relaxed and calm

Let relaxation happen in body and mind

Let it happen

Letting attention dwell easily on body parts, visualizing each part, letting go from tension, starting with feet

Right foot feeling heavy and relaxed

Right foot feeling heavy and relaxed

Left foot feeling heavy and relaxed

Left foot feeling heavy and relaxed

Right ankle feeling heavy and relaxed

Right ankle feeling heavy and relaxed

Left ankle feeling heavy and relaxed

Left ankle feeling heavy and relaxed

Right calf feeling heavy and relaxed

Right calf feeling heavy and relaxed

Left calf feeling heavy and relaxed

Left calf feeling heavy and relaxed

Right knee feeling heavy and relaxed

Right knee feeling heavy and relaxed

Left knee feeling heavy and relaxed

Left knee feeling heavy and relaxed

Right thigh feeling heavy and relaxed
Right thigh feeling heavy and relaxed
Left thigh feeling heavy and relaxed
Left thigh feeling heavy and relaxed
Right hip and buttock feeling heavy and relaxed
Right hip and buttock feeling heavy and relaxed
Left hip and buttock feeling heavy and relaxed
Left hip and buttock feeling heavy and relaxed
Right leg from foot to hip feeling heavy and relaxed
Right leg from foot to hip feeling heavy and relaxed
Left leg from foot to hip feeling heavy and relaxed
Left leg from foot to hip feeling heavy and relaxed
Belly below navel and solar plexus above navel feeling
  comfortable and relaxed
Belly below navel and solar plexus above naval feeling
  comfortable and relaxed
Lower back feeling heavy and relaxed
Lower back feeling heavy and relaxed
Chest muscles feeling comfortable and relaxed
Chest muscles feeling comfortable and relaxed
Breathing deeply and easily
Breathing deeply and easily
Ribs feeling free and·relaxed
Ribs feeling free and relaxed
Belly and solar plexus feeling comfortable and relaxed
Belly and solar plexus feeling comfortable and relaxed
Upper back feeling heavy and relaxed
Upper back feeling heavy and relaxed
Right hand feeling heavy and relaxed
Right hand feeling heavy and relaxed
Left hand feeling heavy and relaxed
Left hand feeling heavy and relaxed
Right forearm feeling heavy and relaxed
Right forearm feeling heavy and relaxed
Left forearm feeling heavy and relaxed
Left forearm feeling heavy and relaxed
Right elbow feeling heavy and relaxed

Right elbow feeling heavy and relaxed
Left elbow feeling heavy and relaxed
Left elbow feeling heavy and relaxed
Right upper arm feeling heavy and relaxed
Right upper arm feeling heavy and relaxed
Left upper arm feeling heavy and relaxed
Left upper arm feeling heavy and relaxed
Right shoulder feeling heavy and relaxed
Right shoulder feeling heavy and relaxed
Left shoulder feeling heavy and relaxed
Left shoulder feeling heavy and relaxed
Right arm from hand to shoulder feeling heavy and relaxed
Right arm from hand to shoulder feeling heavy and relaxed
Left arm from hand to shoulder feeling heavy and relaxed
Left arm from hand to shoulder feeling heavy and relaxed
Right hand feeling relaxed and becoming warm
Right hand feeling relaxed and becoming warm
Warmth flowing into right hand
Warmth flowing into right hand
Right hand feeling warm and relaxed
Right hand feeling warm and relaxed
Left hand feeling relaxed and becoming warm
Left hand feeling relaxed and becoming warm
Warmth flowing into left hand
Warmth flowing into left hand
Left hand feeling warm and relaxed
Left hand feeling warm and relaxed
Right hand in warm sunlight
Left hand in warm sunlight
Passively aware of warmth in the hands
Passively aware of warmth in the hands
Letting warmth come
Letting warmth come
Warmth flowing up right arm
Warmth flowing up right arm
Right lower arm feeling warm and relaxed
Right lower arm feeling warm and relaxed

Warmth flowing up left arm
Warmth flowing up left arm
Left lower arm feeling warm and relaxed
Left lower arm feeling warm and relaxed
Warmth flowing through right elbow into upper arm
Warmth flowing through right elbow into upper arm
Right upper arm feeling warm and relaxed
Right upper arm feeling warm and relaxed
Warmth flowing through left elbow into upper arm
Warmth flowing through left elbow into upper arm
Left upper arm feeling warm and relaxed
Left upper arm feeling warm and relaxed
Warmth flowing into right shoulder
Warmth flowing into right shoulder
Right shoulder feeling warm and relaxed
Right shoulder feeling warm and relaxed
Warmth flowing into left shoulder
Warmth flowing into left shoulder
Left shoulder feeling warm and relaxed
Left shoulder feeling warm and relaxed
Right arm from hand to shoulder feeling warm and relaxed
Right arm from hand to shoulder feeling warm and relaxed
Left arm from hand to shoulder feeling warm and relaxed
Left arm from hand to shoulder feeling warm and relaxed
Feeling relaxed and peaceful
Feeling relaxed and peaceful
Pulse calm and strong
Pulse calm and strong
Feeling relaxed and peaceful
Feeling relaxed and peaceful
Pulse calm and strong
Pulse calm and strong
Warmth reaching all parts of the body
Warmth reaching all parts of the body
Warmth from shoulders flowing into chest and upper back
Warmth from shoulders flowing into chest and upper back
Chest feeling warm and relaxed

Chest feeling warm and relaxed
Upper back feeling warm and relaxed
Upper back feeling warm and relaxed
Breathing calm and regular
Breathing calm and regular
Passively aware of breathing
Passively aware of breathing
Breathing freely
Breathing freely
Breathing calm and regular
Breathing calm and regular
Letting breathing happen
Letting breathing happen
Breathing muscles free and relaxed
Breathing muscles free and relaxed
Letting breathing happen
Letting breathing happen
Being breathed
Being breathed
Breathing calm and relaxed
Breathing calm and relaxed
Warmth flowing into lower back
Warmth flowing into lower back
Lower back feeling warm and relaxed
Lower back feeling warm and relaxed
Solar plexus becoming warm
Solar plexus becoming warm
Solar plexus sun warm
Solar plexus sun warm
Whole abdomen warm and relaxed
Whole abdomen warm and relaxed
Passively aware and letting warmth happen
Passively aware and letting warmth happen
Solar plexus warm
Solar plexus warm
Whole abdomen warm and relaxed
Whole abdomen warm and relaxed

Warmth flowing into pelvis and hips
Warmth flowing into pelvis and hips
Pelvis and hips warm and relaxed
Pelvis and hips warm and relaxed
Warmth flowing into right thigh
Warmth flowing into right thigh
Right thigh warm and relaxed
Right thigh warm and relaxed
Warmth flowing into left thigh
Warmth flowing into left thigh
Left thigh warm and relaxed
Left thigh warm and relaxed
Warmth flowing through right knee into lower leg
Warmth flowing through right knee into lower leg
Right lower leg warm and relaxed
Right lower leg warm and relaxed
Warmth flowing through left knee into lower leg
Warmth flowing through left knee into lower leg
Left lower leg warm and relaxed
Left lower leg warm and relaxed
Warmth flowing through right ankle into foot
Warmth flowing through right ankle into foot
Right foot warm and relaxed
Right foot warm and relaxed
Warmth flowing through left ankle into foot
Warmth flowing through left ankle into foot
Left foot warm and relaxed
Left foot warm and relaxed
Right leg from foot to hip warm and relaxed
Right leg from foot to hip warm and relaxed
Left leg from foot to hip warm and relaxed
Left leg from foot to hip warm and relaxed
Pelvis and abdomen warm and relaxed
Pelvis and abdomen warm and relaxed
Solar plexus warm and relaxed
Solar plexus warm and relaxed
Lower back warm and relaxed

Lower back warm and relaxed
Chest muscles warm and relaxed
Chest muscles warm and relaxed
Upper back warm and relaxed
Upper back warm and relaxed
Right arm from hand to shoulder warm and relaxed
Right arm from hand to shoulder warm and relaxed
Left arm from hand to shoulder warm and relaxed
Left arm from hand to shoulder warm and relaxed
Throat and neck becoming warm and relaxed
Throat and neck becoming warm and relaxed
Whole body from feet to neck feeling warm and relaxed
Whole body from feet to neck feeling warm and relaxed
Warm and relaxed
Warm and relaxed
Mind becoming calm and quiet
Mind becoming calm and quiet
Speech muscles relaxed and still
Speech muscles relaxed and still
Vision muscles relaxed and still
Vision muscles relaxed and still
Mind quiet and serene
Mind quiet and serene
Body and mind still and calm
Body and mind still and calm
Forehead pleasantly cool
Forehead pleasantly cool
Mind cool and calm
Mind cool and calm
Face muscles relaxed
Face muscles relaxed
Body warm and relaxed
Body warm and relaxed
Body in warm sunlight, head in cool shade
Body in warm sunlight, head in cool shade
Pleasant warm sunshine, refreshing cool shade
Pleasant warm sunshine, refreshing cool shade

Arms, legs, and trunk heavy, warm, and relaxed
Arms, legs, and trunk heavy, warm, and relaxed
Head pleasantly cool
Head pleasantly cool
Mind cool and calm
Mind cool and calm
Attention turning inwards
Attention turning inwards
Passively aware of mind relaxed and calm
Passively aware of mind relaxed and calm
Forehead pleasantly cool
Forehead pleasantly cool
Mind cool, calm, and peaceful
Mind cool, calm, and peaceful
Ready to return now to full wakefulness
Ready to return now to full wakefulness
Energy filling arms, legs, and whole body
Energy filling arms, legs, and whole body
All heaviness going
All heaviness going
Facial muscles relaxed and alive
Facial muscles relaxed and alive
Full wakefulness returning on counting back from five to zero
Full wakefulness returning on counting back from five to zero
Five – stretching legs and letting go
Four – stretching arms and letting go
Three – stretching arms and legs and letting go
Two – taking a deep breath and letting it out like a sigh
One – opening eyes, awake, relaxed, and feeling well
Zero – awake and refreshed, sitting up slowly, yawning and
    stretching

## THERAPY AND SELF-IMPROVEMENT

Autogenic training developed out of the uses of auto-suggestion and hypnosis in the treatment of emotional and psychosomatic problems. It is now taught in clinics, sanatoria and rest homes in Germany, Switzerland, Austria, and other parts of Europe and increasingly, psychiatrists in Britain and the USA are using it. It is also one of the methods used by practitioners of 'fringe' or 'alternative' medicine. But almost any person can use autogenic training as a self-help relaxation method and take the opportunity in the deep relaxation state to give positive suggestions for improved health, confidence, changing harmful habits and other forms of self-improvement, just as one might with self-hypnosis.

Schultz wrote of a result claimed from the practice of autogenic training that he called 'the organismic shift', which he said was common to all trainees. Its main features are a state of optimal relaxation and a harmonious functioning of the body as a biological unity that is recognized by trainees through their subjective experiences. There is a feeling of centering, of body and mind as one. This feeling of unity and wellbeing is sustained without the mind being overtaken by distracting thoughts or disrupting emotions; nor is there any slackness or drift into torpor.

It seems to me that Schultz in talking about 'the organismic shift' was describing in his own way the 'relaxation response' given detailed scientific investigation by Dr Herbert Benson about fifty years later.

Autogenic training gives all the benefits associated with the relaxation response – release of stress, deep physiological rest, renewal of energies, enhanced concentration, clarity of consciousness, and so on.

Because autogenic training heightens sensitivity to body sensations and physiological processes, it is not considered a suitable therapy for psychotics or hypochondriacs or any person already paying obsessive or neurotic attention to their body perceptions. But for the majority of people, withdrawing from external impressions and becoming aware of impressions from within is helpful, for to have such sensitive awareness is the beginning of the possibility of control. Most people can learn to calm heartbeat and breathing, reduce blood pressure, improve blood circulation and direct warmth and thoughts of healing to unhealthy or damaged body parts.

Painful areas of the body can be given immediate relief through relaxation and passive awareness, which dissolve tension and release the grip of contracted muscles that cause pain. Another reason they give relief is that you are no longer adding to the pain by having painful thoughts about pain – you are just aware and nothing more! Warmth also soothes pain and aids healing, and autogenics develops skill in increasing the temperature of selected body areas. In very cold conditions, this skill can be used to bring comfort to the body and prevent hands and feet feeling frozen. The Tibetan Yogins greatly develop this skill – which they call *tumo* – and may meditate for hours, wearing only light clothing, in mountain temperatures well below zero.

Autogenics develops a capacity to withstand severe stress. Dr Hannes Lindemann crossed the Atlantic Ocean alone in an open boat and wrote afterwards that he could not have succeeded in so arduous an enterprise but for the self-mastery he had built up through the practice of autogenic training.

Doctors at the Menninger Clinic in America have combined autogenic training with biofeedback to teach sufferers from migraine to induce warmth in their hands and coolness in their foreheads. Two thirds of these patients reported relief of head pains.

For more than fifty years autogenic training has been used in Europe for the treatment of psychosomatic and tension disorders. Progressive relaxation has been used in America for about the same period and for the same purposes. The quasi-mystical vagueness of language used by some European operators of autogenic training has perhaps delayed its incorporation into general medical practice in England and the USA; but then it is only recently that hypnosis has thrown off its 'exotic' image and been accepted in the same conservative quarters. Increasingly, progressive relaxation and autogenic training are being combined as therapies, and both combined with biofeedback – the use of machines to monitor such 'hidden' internal processes as brain wave rhythms, temperature, blood pressure, and so on. That will be the subject of the following chapter.

# 6 Biofeedback

Biofeedback was developed by medical scientists in the United States in the 1960s. as a guided self-help therapy. Biofeedback instruments are useful in monitoring and aiding progress in muscular and mental relaxation, and relaxation therapy is a major part of biofeedback therapy. The kind of ailments and behavioural problems treated by biofeedback are largely those treated by other forms of relaxation therapy.

Unfortunately, the best instruments are as yet expensive for purchase for individual home use, and access to instruments is not yet widely available. Perhaps one day there will be relaxation centres in most towns and cities making biofeedback technology available to the general public.

## WHAT IS BIOFEEDBACK?

Biofeedback is the technical term used to describe the instrumental monitoring of one's biological functions for the purpose of gaining control over them. Or, to put it another way: biofeedback is the voluntary control of what were formerly thought to be involuntary psychophysiological states, achieved through the use of electronic instruments monitoring the states.

Control is gained through a learning process based on visible, auditory, or other signals telling the subject what is going on inside him or her. The signals are objective correlates of inner physiological processes whose changes correspond to changes made by the subject exercising self-control. Most people, after a few hours of biofeedback training, achieve levels of control over processes normally operated only by the autonomic nervous system. Hitherto this kind of control was accredited only to yogins, shamans, and other people said to have extraordinary powers (*siddhis*).

Electronic biofeedback gives opportunities for control over muscle tension and relaxation, blood pressure, heart rate, and even brainwave rhythms, including those associated with states of consciousness linked with the practice of meditation and with mystical development. Many people are drawn to biofeedback as a meditation aid and others as a relaxation therapy.

Reliance on the machines need only be temporary. The aim of biofeedback training is to make the subject independent of the instrument once skill in self-control has been developed. The capacity to change bodily and mental states is usually long-lasting, and the instruments may be used for 'refresher' training at any time.

## LEARNING RELAXATION

The sensitivity of biofeedback instruments in signalling the presence of muscle tension difficult for the subject to detect makes biofeedback an excellent aid to learning to relax. We easily habituate to states of tension and think that by lying or sitting motionless and comfortable we are free of tension. Biofeedback technology exposes that fallacy.

Biofeedback is useful in speeding up the time taken to learn deep psychophysical relaxation. It both tests progress in relaxation and gives training in the awareness required to let go further from tension. Degrees of tension and relaxation in muscles in any part of the body can be measured. Other instruments signal the presence in the brain of electrical wave rhythms linked with mental relaxation and meditation consciousness.

# THE INSTRUMENTS

We are only concerned here with the instruments that relate to learning bodily and mental relaxation.

The electromyograph (EMG) monitors the electrical activity produced in muscles by the firing of motor neurons in muscle action or tension. It pinpoints areas of the body where tension is prone to develop and persist. It is used in the treatment of physical and mental problems caused by or accompanied by excessive muscle tension. The muscles selected for monitoring in therapy are those most likely to be tensed. The *frontalis* muscle of the forehead is often selected for biofeedback treatment of tension headaches and anxiety states.

Another way to measure states of tension and of absence of tension (relaxation) is through skin resistance to an electrical current passed through it. High resistance indicates relaxation, low resistance indicates tension. Electrical skin resistance (ESR) machines record levels of arousal and non-arousal in the fingertips or in the palms of the hands. The range of use is not so great as with EMG equipment.

The temperature meter measures the temperature of selected skin areas and leads to control of skin temperature. Warmth in the hand and coolness in the forehead has relevance to the practice of autogenic relaxation and to the treatment of tension headaches, Raynaud's syndrome and some other disorders.

The electroencephalogram (EEG) monitors brainwave rhythms. Because of the interest in alpha waves, some lower-priced machines indicate alpha activity only. Moving the eyes, forehead, or other facial muscles may produce alpha waves, so in using EEG equipment it is important to keep the face relaxed and motionless.

British scientist Maxwell Cade has developed the 'mind mirror', which converts the signals from the brain's two cortical hemispheres into an illuminated display making visible a total pattern formation.

# BRAIN WAVE RHYTHMS

For EEG monitoring of brainwave rhythms, electrodes are placed at various points on the scalp. The main rhythms to keep in mind are the fast frequency beta, 13–30 Hz, alpha 8–12 Hz, theta 4–7 Hz, and delta ½–4 Hz.

Biofeedback enables us to look at our midbrain in a new way, both seeing and experiencing its complexity. It shows that human emotions, forms of attention and mental activities have their characteristic brainwave frequencies, amplitudes and patterns.

Beta activity is associated with the performance of physical and mental tasks, but if the task has become easy it may be performed with alpha rhythms in the brain. Albert Einstein was said to be able to solve difficult arithmetical problems while producing predominant alpha in his brain.

Alpha waves of low frequency are associated with states of deep relaxation, with reverie and with rest immediately following concentrated mental effort. They are also characteristic of attention passively dwelling on internal events or on external events where what is observed is stabilized, as in gazing at a flower, landscape, or seascape, following a moving object with a steady swing of the gaze, and so on. This links alpha with the practice of meditation, and Maxwell Cade and other researchers associate alpha activity in the brain with meditation or fourth state consciousness. The first three states are dreamless sleep, dreaming sleep and ordinary waking consciousness.

Most people find the alpha experience pleasant and relaxing. Volunteers are never lacking for alpha research programmes. A leading American researcher, Elmer Green, has described the alpha feeling as 'passive volition'. This ties up with the 'effortless concentration', 'choiceless awareness', 'creative passivity', 'action that is non-action', and so on of Eastern types of tranquillity meditation. Passive volition could also describe the state of mind needed for learning the relaxation methods described in earlier chapters of this book.

In 1958, Dr Joe Kamiya, a psychologist investigating sleep states, made the discovery that his subjects could produce alpha waves at will by relating to an auditory signal that let them know when their brains were in alpha. Independently, Dr Barbara B. Brown, now a prominent writer and lecturer on the biofeedback 'revolution', was training subjects to produce alpha waves with open eyes, which is more difficult than with eyes closed. A blue light illuminated when alpha was produced and intensified or dimmed according to the largeness or smallness of the waves in the brain.

The even slower theta rhythm is also associated with reverie and with meditation, and is particularly linked with dreaming and the half-sleep states entering and coming out of sleep.

The extremely slow delta rhythm is mainly associated with deep, dreamless sleep. Some investigators link it with the onset of paranormal phenomena.

## BIOFEEDBACK AND MEDITATION

Studies of Japanese Zen, Indian Yogin, American, British and other meditators show that in meditation consciousness there is predominant slow alpha activity when the mind is calm. If there is an upsurge of devotional or other ecstasy, beta then occurs. There is some theta activity in deep meditation states.

Maxwell Cade's mind mirror records symmetrical patterns across the brain's two hemispheres. Some researchers see the left and right hemispheres as representing two contrasting modes of consciousness.

Left hemisphere functioning could be summed up as rational consciousness. It is concerned with logical, linear, step-by-step thinking, with speech, with time sense, with analytical tasks, such as categorizing and naming what we see.

Right hemisphere functioning could be summed up as intuitive or aesthetic consciousness. It is concerned with intuition, holism, recognizing wholes or *Gestalts* (for example, faces), spatial and musical relationships, such as are necessary for painting, sculpting and dancing. It is non-linear and non-verbal.

Left hemisphere thinking is typical of Western culture and right hemisphere thinking of Eastern culture. The practice of meditation and the cultivation of Oriental attitudes will, according to this approach, develop right hemisphere functioning.

Progress in poised living comes gradually. Daily 'dips' into deep relaxation lead to increasing ability to be relaxed and mentally calm in all aspects of living. This is one of the main goals of the practice of meditation, our fifth and final method for eliciting the relaxation response. But before describing practical meditation techniques, it is necessary to consider two essential preparations for the practice of meditation which are in themselves expressions of relaxed living – poised posture and poised breathing.

# 7 *Poised Posture and Poised Breathing*

## POSTURE AND PSYCHOPHYSICAL WELLBEING

The way the body is held and used has a most important bearing on its health and efficiency. If the body is carried well and harmoniously balanced, muscular work will be performed with the minimum of fatigue. Poor posture, on the other hand, will cramp the muscles, impose a strain on the joints and impair the proper functioning of the internal organs.

L. Jean Bogert, in *Nutrition and Physical Fitness*, explains:

Bad posture may put certain parts of the body under strain or cramp them so that the blood supply to them is poor and they are unable to do their work effectively. A deep chest of potentially large air capacity may actually produce poorer aeration of the blood, if held in a cramped position and supported by a low and flabby diaphragm muscle so that breathing is shallow, than a chest of lesser capacity which is used with maximum efficiency. A stomach which is capable of doing its job well when in normal position may give constant trouble when it has sagged so far down in the abdomen that its contents may be emptied against gravity or its blood and nerve supply are interfered with. An intestine which formerly functioned well may lose the good tone of its muscle wall when there is habitual stagnation of its blood supply, due to its position in the abdomen and to the inactivity of the diaphragm, which is largely responsible for 'milking' the blood out of the abdomen back toward the heart by its rhythmic contractions in breathing.

Thus we see that right posture and right breathing go together.

In good posture the abdominal cavity is pear-shaped with its larger end uppermost, fitting comfortably into the natural position between the ribs. In poor posture a flat chest plus sagging ribs force the viscera down and out until the shape of the abdominal cavity is the reverse of that in the normal healthy position; the pear shape remains, but now the narrower end is on top.

Poised use of the body prevents fatigue and wear and tear; poor mechanical use causes unnecessary tiredness and aches and pains in muscles and joints. Good body use is conducive to body–mind harmony and a feeling of poised and effortless living that some people can equate with the flow of life, or, as the Chinese say, the Tao.

By bringing balance and poise to our physical selves we induce these same valuable qualities in our psychical selves. This total harmony is better understood and more keenly sought in the East than in the West.

Emotional excitement increases our rate of respiration. By breathing slowly and smoothly we calm the emotions.

To attain spiritual poise the Eastern adept trains his (or her) body to be relaxed and poised. He breathes slowly and rhythmically, and stills his mind by awareness of his breathing or by practising some other form of meditation.

## COMMON POSTURAL FAULTS

1  The head too far forward or too far back
2  The head inclined slightly to one side
3  The head turned slightly to one side
4  The chin held high or low instead of level
5  One shoulder held lower than the other shoulder
6  One shoulder twisted around
7  The shoulders hunched forward, cramping the chest: the hollow chest
8  The shoulders pulled back too far: the pouter pigeon chest
9  The shoulders raised; often a sign of tension

10  A rounded upper back
11  A hollowed lower back
12  The hips too far foward or too far back, instead of balanced
    on the central invisible line around which the body weight
    should be properly distributed
13  Bodyweight too much on the heels or on the balls of the
    feet, instead of being evenly distributed over both feet.

The most common postural fault is a round back or *kyphosis*,
which is often due to carrying the head forward, exerting harmful pressure on the upper spine where it joins to the skull. Short-
sighted people may develop a round back through pressing
forward frequently with the head; faulty seating, poor lighting
and overwork are other causes. Bending the head forward over
work, instead of keeping the head, neck and back in alignment,
causes a round back with attendant strains on the lower back as
well as on the upper vertebrae. Hollow back or *lordosis* is most
often seen in young children and may persist into adult life.

## POSTURE IN CHILDREN

Most infants display excellent posture. Note the way most
toddlers keep head and back in line when picking up an object
from the floor. But by the age of five or six postural faults have
already appeared in many children.

Postural training should be part of the curriculum in
Western schools from primary level, but it is rarely included.

Jack Vinten Fenton, an English headmaster with knowledge
of the Alexander method of postural training, wrote an excellent guide on teaching body mechanics to schoolchildren, with
the title *Choice of Habit*. In the book he tells of two six month
projects in postural re-education at a primary and at a secondary
school. Both projects were successful in discovering postural
faults in pupils and in tackling them. Stoops and hollow backs
were corrected, raised shoulders were brought down, and so
on. Holding up the shoulders is a frequent sign of tension. The
shoulders should hang loosely: when they do, the arm move-

ments required for calisthenics, sports and games become freer and more efficient.

Through postural training, one boy obtained relief from asthma and another boy from stammering; both boys were at primary school. Teachers at the secondary school reported increased efficiency in pupils during cookery and art classes. A teacher reported: 'In art both girls and boys are making pictures full of movement. This has shown real application backed by the excellent teaching of the art mistress where the understanding of a forward and upward direction of the spine is reflected in the work.' This principle of 'upward release' is an important part of the Alexander method.

An interesting project for the secondary school pupils was collecting cuttings from newspapers and magazines showing children and adults of all ages standing, sitting or engaged in various activities. The pupils were also encouraged to collect pictures of people of different races and from different periods in history. They were told to study the pictures and see what could be learned about the effects on people's posture of environment, age, furniture and any other influences.

If the collected pictures included any of women in India or Africa carrying pitchers on their heads, or of meditating Yogins or Buddhist monks, then superb models of what is entailed in poised posture would have been illustrated.

For wrong and harmful postures, the schoolchildren could not have done better than find photographs of the training of cadets at West Point in the USA. Rigidity and tension are often considered an essential part of training fighting men in the West, and the postures adopted are often those in which one would expect a slow reaction for any call to instant action. Comparing the Western military posture with the relaxed yet alert posture of the experienced exponent of judo or *kendo* or any Eastern martial arts reveals much about Eastern and Western attitudes.

The schoolchildren in these projects were encouraged to check their postures in mirrors and to assist each other by observing postural faults or praising correct body use.

More teaching of correct body use to schoolchildren would lead to greater efficiency in sports, games, woodwork, cookery, art, and in writing and reading. Brainwork also might improve, for the brain is likely to be better oxygenated.

## THREE POSTURES

It is important to understand that if poor posture has become habitual, then right posture is going to feel 'wrong' at first. The strangeness of the new posture lasts a few days, until the new feeling of body poise has become familiar.

Check progress in a full-length mirror, standing sideways and swinging your eyes across to look, having turned your head as little as possible. Thereby you can observe any faults and check that your posture is approaching and finally sustaining healful poise. A mirror provides visual feedback, a concept that was discussed in the preceding chapter. A friend who himself or herself learns poised posture can also help point out adjustments that may be necessary in body use.

Now we come to a most important point. Good posture is not a matter of pulling parts of your body in or pushing other parts out, which leads only to a temporary approximation of physical poise, but is more a matter of new *thinking*. Thinking mainly as sensed image, though in the early days of postural training verbal formulae can be helpful.

The key to posture control is relaxing the neck and 'thinking' upwards with the head, with the spine easing up from the lead of the head. With conscious attention to this for a time, poised posture eventually becomes habitual.

That the head is the primary control was the key discovery of F. Matthias Alexander, founder of the Alexander method of postural training. Carrying a pitcher on your head achieves a similar effect, though could be viewed as eccentricity by friends and neighbours if put into practice. The crosslegged sitting postures of Eastern meditators also induces the right feeling of poise. Readers may make a radical improvement in posture if attention is given to the two practical measures just mentioned:

lightly poising the head on the spine while thinking 'upwards', and sitting for meditation, especially in one of the traditional positions.

But first let us construct a mental picture of what is required through considering three basic upright postures that one can observe in others. The first two postures are common but harmful. The third posture is our goal of poised posture, and in many ways finds a golden mean between the other two harmful postures, which I call 'slumped posture' and 'rigid posture'.

Remember that right posture leads to right breathing, the muscles of respiration being unconstricted and able to function easily.

## SLUMPED POSTURE

This posture is frequently seen. The head and whole body sags and slumps. The upper back is rounded and the lower back is hollowed. The head juts forward, which is the primary problem. Reasons why this may happen have been given above.

The chest slumps and flattens, and the belly collapses its tone and protrudes. The upper body presses down on the protruding abdomen and its internal organs. Because the considerable weight of the head is carried too far forward in relation to the pelvis, the spine is bent like a bow, matching the hump of the upper back and the hollow curve of the lower back. The leg muscles and hip and leg joints strain to support the imbalanced structure above them.

Many body muscles are unnecessarily tensed to cope with the chain of imbalances descending from the forward weight of the head. Aches and pains are frequent and spinal problems are likely to arise.

Because this posture may to the untrained eye look slack, it would be wrong to think there is anything easygoing about it. A slumped posture entails unnecessary effort to sustain it in work, play or rest. It is sloppy and inefficient. It represents a partial collapse and body muscles that should not have to work so hard or even work at all are fighting to prevent total collapse. The slumped posture represents strain, not relaxation.


## RIGID POSTURE

This might have been called military posture, but, as already pointed out, it represents a strange idea of what is required in a man of action.

This is in many ways the opposite of the slumped posture, but represents an excess of its own that maintains tension unnecessarily and therefore a superfluous expenditure of energy. Compared with slumped posture, there is overcompensation and overcorrection.

The chin is pulled back and the neck is shortened and contracted, squeezing on nerves passing from the spinal column to the brain, interfering with blood supply, and pressing the skull down on the upper vertebrae.

The uplifted and thrust out chest does not indicate better breathing, because it means that only the upper parts of the lungs are used and relaxed healthy breathing is prevented. The breathing muscles are kept contracted and do not have the relaxed mobility needed for efficient bellows-like contraction and expansion by the lungs.

In rigid posture the chin is often raised, so that the head is pulled back and the spine from top to bottom is compressed. The bottom juts and the pelvis is carried too far back instead of being tucked in and upward.

The body is tensed, strained and under pressure.


## POISED POSTURE

Body parts in easy, natural balance.

The body expanded, poised, alert, ready for instant action.

The neck is relaxed and the head lightly poised on the spine.

The head and the spine ease upwards to initiate and carry out movement.

The chin is held level. To tilt the head down or back, think of a hinge at the ear and not at the neck.

The head, neck and spine are in alignment.

Think of an invisible line drawn from the top of your head, down through your body to your feet. Bodyweight in poised posture is evenly distributed about this invisible line so that the skeleton, ligaments and major muscle groups bear the proportionate load allocated by nature. Under such natural arrangement the limbs and muscles work in an efficient and economical way.

Poised posture begins with the head. The head is the primary control from which the rest should follow. Poise the head easily on the neck as a flower on its stalk.

The spine is free to ease upward, not curved forward as in the slumped posture or compressed as in the rigid posture. There is a sense of lengthening and broadening in the back. The arms and legs, too, feel as though they are lengthening. The thought or sense is of the head moving upwards and the trunk following.

The shoulders hang loose and low.

The ribs feel free to move in and out and the diaphragm to move down and up in easy respiration. The abdomen is released to swell out slightly as the diaphragm moves down and flattens back towards the spine slightly as the diaphragm moves up.

The upper body feels up and out of the hips.

The abdomen feels flat and firm compared with the collapse of tone in the slumped posture, but the belly has a natural release and a gentle curve to it that contrasts with the contrived pulling back of the rigid posture.

The bodyweight is evenly distributed over both legs and feet.

There is a sense of lightness and buoyancy, of making light of gravity.

## POSTURE AND PERSONALITY

Physical posture influences mental posture, just as inner posture influences outer posture.

Each of the three basic postures described above reveals a

tendency for psychological traits to match up with the physical characteristics of the posture. This does not amount to every person displaying each posture having the personality factors listed below. But there is a propensity to have or to develop them. This amounts to saying that improving posture could be a method of self-improvement. In the East, poised posture is taught as a psychotherapy as well as a main technique of spiritual unfoldment.

*Slumped posture*

| | | |
|---|---|---|
| apathy | gravity | melancholy |
| awkwardness | grief | sag |
| boredom | heaviness | slackness |
| clumsiness | heaviness of heart | sloppiness |
| dejection | indifference | slowness |
| depression | inefficiency | sluggishness |
| drag | jadedness | slump |
| droop | lethargy | staleness |
| drooping spirits | lifelessness | tiredness |
| fatigue | low | weakness |
| flatness | low spirits | weariness |
| gloom | | |

*Rigid posture*

| | | |
|---|---|---|
| aggression | harshness | repression |
| anger | impatience | rigorousness |
| clench | impenetrability | severity |
| constipation | inflexibility | sternness |
| defensiveness | intolerance | stiffness |
| dogmatism | irascibility | strain |
| excitability | militancy | stubbornness |
| fanaticism | nonfluidity | tenseness |
| fear | ossification | tension |
| fixedness | petrification | tightness |
| fright | rage | unyieldingness |
| hardness | | |

*Poised posture*

absorption
alertness
attention
awareness
balance
beauty
being
calmness
centring
clarity
compassion
composure
concentration
contemplation
coolness
detachment
dignity
ease
efficiency
enlightenment
equanimity

equilibrium
equipoise
gracefulness
harmony
imperturbability
letting go
love
lucidity
meditation
mindfulness
moderation
non-attachment
openness
order
peace
peacefulness
poise
quiet
quietude
relaxation
repose

rest
self-actualization
self-command
self-control
self-possession
self-realization
sensitivity
serenity
smoothness
softness (overcoming
hard, like water)
stability
steadiness
stillness
suppleness
symmetry
tolerance
tranquillity
unflappability
*wu wei* (Chinese,
not forcing,
not striving

## HARA, OR BELLY WISDOM

On the principle that outer influences inner, just as inner influences outer, poised posture has a prominent place in Eastern culture. This is particularly true of Japanese culture, in which there is considerable Zen influence.

Poised posture has an essential role in the practice of such arts as calligraphy, ink painting, pottery, puppetry, Noh acting, the tea ceremony and flower arranging. It is also basic to such sports (and arts) as archery, aikido, judo, kendo (swordsmanship) and sumo wrestling.

Sitting in poised posture is the physical basis for the practice of meditation in Zen and in other schools of Buddhism, and is st the whole of meditation in one school of Zen, the *Soto*.

For right posture to play its full role it has to serve right inner posture, a Zen attitude based on full awareness of the present moment, mindfulness, spontaneity, mental clarity, the healthful interplay of positive and negative, *yang* and *yin* forces in the body, with no interference from the petty ego-self with its thoughts of success and failure, profit and loss.

Posture and breathing in Japanese culture and in meditation are linked with the concept and practice known as *hara*.

Hara is the Japanese word for 'belly', but has a significance that goes far beyond the literal meaning. Philip Kapleau, in *Zen: Dawn in the West*, says:

In Zen, the hara – or more correctly the tanden, which is specifically the lower abdomen – is recognized as the body–mind's vital centre, and by learning to focus the mind there and to radiate all one's activities from that region, one develops greater mental and physical equilibrium and a reserve of energy.

The term hara takes in the abdomen from the stomach down to the lower belly. The *tanden*, considered to be the body's exact centre of gravity, is precisely located: about two inches below the navel.

*Haragei* is the Japanese name for the art of hara, which can be applied in a variety of artistic, ritualistic and sporting activities. These activities are judged by the discerning onlooker not so much for the end results *per se* but for what they tell us about the state of consciousness of the artist, the ritualist and the sportsman.

In Japan, arts, crafts and sports are looked upon as forms of spiritual training. There is a Way of Archery, a Way of Swordsmanship, a Way of Wrestling, a Way of Self-defence, a Way of Tea-Drinking, a Way of Calligraphy, a Way of Pottery-Making and so on. These activities are ways of training in Zen. Poised posture and poised breathing, centred in hara, provide the physical basis of these arts that are also ways, influencing and being influenced by the mental states and stances or inner posture and breathing of Zen.

Hara is the focus for the instinctive wisdom of the body–mind, the power and intelligence of the unconscious. It is the whole person in his liaison with the vital energies within him. The person centred in hara has superb balance and poise, yet at the same time seems rooted in the earth. The person with hara is literally no pushover. The art of hara is demonstrated both by the power and nimbleness of the huge sumo wrestler and the precision and spontaneity of the artist with his brush and ink.

Eugen Herrigel studied Zen in Japan and was advised to follow the Way of Archery. His account of his years of training with a master archer has become a modern classic of Zen literature for westerners. His training was not just in a sport but in an inner discipline. The master, Kenzo Awa, had an extremely powerful bow that only he could pull. He pulled it with an arm whose muscles stayed soft and relaxed. He explained that it was not necessary to make any effort when drawing the bow. What was required was to stand in poised posture, breathe well, centre the body and awareness in the lower belly, relax the arm muscles, and 'pull within the mind'.

In aikido one adopts the posture of *ten-chi* (sky and earth) – that is, the posture of perfect balance. Similarly in archery, the master tells the pupil to think of the top of the bow as piercing the sky and the bottom as piercing the earth. The really important thing is not for the arrow to hit the centre of the target, though this may be accomplished, but for the arrow to shoot by itself. The archer does not shoot. 'It' shoots. Ego and intention have dropped away. Professor Herrigel was told: 'It is something, not yourself, which draws the bow.' Success is measured by how far the archer is able to step aside from his ego, and is only indirectly related to a scoring system. This is a strange concept to the average Western sportsman; but in recent years books have been published in America on how the Zen attitude can bring improvement and greater fulfilment in tennis, golf, running and other sports.

The Zen approach is the same, whatever sport is chosen as a

In judo and aikido the force used by an opponent is converted into victorious use by submitting to it and then taking advantage of the opponent's momentum or lack of balance. An excellent example of effectively following the Tao or way of least resistance.

Hara gives a reliable physical base to posture; the psycho-physical energies are gathered together in the lower belly. 'Upright, firm, and collected' sum up the Japanese view of good posture. The Japanese do not find a large belly ugly if it belongs to a person in hara, but size is not the issue. In Japanese posture the lower belly is released yet firm, and the size of the belly is not important.

Training aimed at perfecting any skill or art can be training in an 'inner way'. Thus a trade can be work on the inner way if the attitude brought to bear on it is the right one. That is why motor cycle maintenance can be training in Zen, a point made in a surprising bestseller by the American Robert M. Pirsig. The Japanese have a saying: 'Archery and dancing, flower-arranging and singing, tea-drinking and wrestling – it is all the same.'

Performance of any skill or art in the Zen view should look spontaneous, easy and natural – the art that conceals art. Great skill is only admired in so far as it reveals inner ripeness and maturity.

Persistent training in an art brings the trainee to the point where the technical skill becomes automatic. Then the ego-self with its constant calculation of profit or loss in terms of self-esteem can be dropped and being itself fills awareness.

Karlfried Graf Von Durckheim, a philosopher and psycho-therapist, has written a book *Hara: The Vital Centre of Man* which shows the considerable influence of hara on Japanese life and culture. He was himself trained in sitting meditation (*zazen*). He shows how hara relates to the Zen practice of 'just sitting', and to realizing creative relaxation and maintaining health. He sees hara as primarily an attitude (*Verfassung*) – 'an all-inclusive general attitude which enables a man to open himself to the power and wholeness of the original life-force and to testify to it by the fulfilment, the meaningfulness and the mastery displayed in his own life.'

Hara is thus seen to have universal validity, though in Japan the practice may be equated with Zen.

Rooting oneself in the vital centre keeps the ego's forces in check. They are not allowed to ignore and separate themselves from nature. Centring in hara is standing in being. As Martin Heidegger pointed out, Westerners are forgetful of being. Centring in hara is a method of discovering or rediscovering being.

The vital centre in man testifies to natural order. Imbalanced posture disrupts and distorts natural order. Relaxation and poise are found through respect for nature and centring in its order.

According to the Zen masters, when the focus of existence is in the belly rather than above it, the body operates with a natural interplay of contraction and relaxation. They say that centring higher than the abdomen is characteristic of ego-control and rigidity of body and mind. The average Westerner is centred in the chest or higher: he is ego hard, imbalanced in body use, has a body–mind split, his conscious and unconscious minds are at war, and he is forgetful of being. Centring in the abdomen, the body's natural centre of gravity, is the Zen way to relaxation and poise, to body–mind unity, to conscious – unconscious harmony, and awareness of being.

Hara posture is important to the Japanese because they see it as a sign of inner maturity: as without, so within. The individual in hara is in-form-ed as a psychophysical whole. To strengthen hara is to increase bodily, mental and spiritual energy.

## STRENGTHENING HARA

Releasing the lower abdomen and putting strength in it is, like the primary control of the Alexander method, a mental rather than a physical act. Thrusting out the abdomen is an erroneous interpretation, and so is tightening the abdominal muscles, just as in the Alexander method one should not go about thrusting one's head upwards. When breathing is naturally deep and into the abdomen, this is in itself a considerable means of strengthening hara. In poised posture deep diaphragmatic and abdominal breathing comes naturally.

There should be no thought of the upper body slumping down. Firm hara supports the upper body and enables it to be relaxed and free and eased upwards with good spinal alignment and separation. Look at photographs of Japanese men or women engaged in meditation or any of the arts I have mentioned and you will see a firm, collected, erect but easy posture in which the head is lightly poised on the neck, and the head, neck and back are in natural alignment.

I believe that the habit from childhood of sitting crosslegged or on their heels on the floor accounts for so many Oriental people having a superior posture to most Occidental people. The Western child is brought up to copy adults and sit on chairs of incredibly foolish design in relation to the shape and health of the human body. The habit of slumping and rounding the back starts early in life and is often established by the ages of five or six years. Hence the need for correction of body posture and use.

Settling in hara is easier to attain when in a sitting posture than in a standing position. This is especially true of crosslegged sitting in any of the traditional meditation postures. Such sitting is worth cultivating by every person who can possibly do so. The full lotus position with both feet upturned on the thighs is difficult for most Westerners, but there are easier positions of symmetrical stability in which the centre of gravity in the lower belly becomes the focus of awareness and in which the human energies can be collected and accumulated.

How to sit in poised posture with poised breathing will be described in the following chapter. Meanwhile note that the perfect embodiment of posture in hara is the meditating Zen monk. There is perfect centring in being. Statues of the serene meditating Buddha display poised sitting posture in metal or stone.

Karl Von Durckheim was taught in Japan to do three things

for right posture: to drop the shoulders, to release the lower belly, and to put strength in the lower belly or tanden. All three stages are achieved without forcing. The shoulders are allowed to drop, not forced down. The lower belly is released, not pushed not. The sustained focus of awareness in the lower belly plus abdominal breathing generates strength in the tanden. The lower abdomen moves forward slightly while the pit of the stomach falls in slightly. The whole trunk above the navel is firm but relaxed, buoyant even. There is a sense of strength and stability below and of freedom above. The new balance of stability and freedom causes changes in personality and one experiences why poised posture is part of an inner way of liberation from ego tensions and conditioning.

When the lower abdomen is released and the upper body is free, the ribs, diaphragm and abdomen function easily in breathing. This is in itself a means of generating energy in the tanden. There is a connection, too, between breathing in the lower belly, quietening the mind and building spiritual energy, which will be explained in the following chapter.

That great physical energy can be gathered and generated in the lower belly is well known in practical ways to experienced athletes who learn how to synchronize their breathing with muscular effort for maximum results. They learn when to take a deep breath, when to let it out, and when and how long to hold a breath before letting it out. This control stems largely from the diaphragm and belly.

The holding of breath at times is important, and not only for the athlete. It is important for the artist making a precise brush-stroke, for the potter throwing a bowl on the wheel, for a singer pausing before attacking a high note, for the surgeon making an incision, as well as for the sprinter about to 'explode' out of the starting blocks. For the circus performer breath control makes the difference between success and failure, perhaps even between life and death.

When a reporter for a Fleet Street national newspaper, I interviewed a footballer famous for his great power in kicking a 'dead' ball. He scored frequently from free kicks, often taken well outside the penalty box. I asked him if he knew the secret of his kicking power. His reply was: 'I wind myself up, take a deep breath, hold it, then explode!' I had not read about Zen and the strength in the tanden in those days and so did not think to ask the footballer what he felt in his lower belly when taking a free kick. But I imagine his answer would have been a concentration of power in that region of the body. It would have arisen from holding his breath and from gathering his energies into a ball as firm as the one he was about to kick. Then the release, the explosion of tightly gathered energy.

The holding of strength in the belly is visible in the experienced weightlifter, just before his final release of breath and explosion of muscular effort. In some countries, such as Egypt, it is customary for weightlifters to shout a dedication of the lift to a past master in the sport just as the breath is released and the barbell hurled overhead. A similar use of the breathing muscles and a powerful shout gives added strength to the exponent of karate, or of judo which I once heard described as 'twist and shout'. Westerners are often amused by the shouts, but they are ignorant of hara.

In karate, in judo, in aikido, in kendo, and in sumo wrestling movements are controlled from the tanden, which is at the same time the source of great physical, mental and spiritual energy. The reason the sumo wrestler squats, feet wide apart, hands on the mat, and stares at his opponent for some time is because this position places his centre of gravity firmly in the lower belly and one-pointed concentration generates energy in the *tanden*, like charging a battery. This may happen five or six times. Breath control is also important. When the sumo wrestler considers he is full of *kiai*, he hurls himself at his opponent. *Ki* literally means 'breath' and *ai* 'to adjust'. Breath is controlled from the tanden.

The relationship between poised posture, breathing, and the lower belly is important not only in Japanese sport and the arts, but also for Zen sitting meditation.

The Japanese speak of *hara no aru hito* and *hara no nai hito* – 'the man with centre' and 'the man without centre'. The man with hara has strength combined with calmness, balance and tranquillity. The man without centre lacks these qualities.

From this discussion of hara it will be clear why the Japanese admire the person who is said to speak from the belly, think from the belly, listen from the belly, and so on.

## THE ALEXANDER METHOD

The West has its own esoteric cult of posture in the Alexander method, which is less well known than hara is in Japan and less accepted generally. This is to a large extent due to the personality of the founder, who, though attracting support from some celebrities, had difficulty in expressing his ideas clearly either for general readers or for the scientific fraternity. One of the supporting celebrities, Aldous Huxley, offered to write for Alexander but the offer was turned down. If the offer had been accepted, it could have done a great deal to popularize the Alexander method. Aldous Huxley does have some things to say about Alexander's postural training and ideas in *Ends and Means* and *Eyeless in Gaza*.

Frederick Matthias Alexander was born in 1869 in the small town of Wynyard in Tasmania. He developed a love of the theatre at an early age and became an actor, specializing in dramatic recitals. But a serious problem arose; during recitals he sometimes lost his voice. Doctors were unable to help and Alexander sought his own cure for what was a terrible professional handicap. He studied himself in mirrors while reciting. It took nine years for him to solve his problem. He noticed that in initiating movements he tended to pull his head backwards and down; this applied to all aspects of living and was part of wrong body use, having the effect of lifting the chest and compressing the spine. This was the cause of his speech problem and, he believed, a chain of postural and health problems that he saw in other people. That a great many people throw back their heads slightly on rising from sitting on a chair is easily observed.

Alexander, through studying his own patterns of body use, thus hit upon what he termed the primary control – the correct positioning of the head in relation to the spine, which is made possible by relaxing the neck. Good posture followed from understanding the primary control.

Alexander went to London where he taught postural training. Eventually he trained some men and women to become instructors in the method. Some of them have, since Alexander's death in London in 1955, said how confusing and slow the training was. Alexander wrote four books through which the reader struggles to come out with no practical instruction. He was clearly reluctant to put practical exercises in print, which has limited the training to a few people able to find a teacher of the method and to pay the fees.

My own sense of frustration and irritation on reading Alexander and some of his followers, who seemed to have the same inhibitory malaise as the founder, must have been duplicated thousands of times. I experience a similar irritation today on reading books about transcendental meditation, which also praise the method but do not come out with any practical instruction; that is reserved for the fee payers. In fact, both the Alexander method and transcendental meditation are very simple techniques that could be described easily in a book. Both are effective and highly beneficial techniques that deserve to reach the mass of the people.

This difficulty with the Alexander method was solved, to my satisfaction, in 1978. In the intervening twenty-five years my pursuit of poised posture had been based on what I saw as two perfect models – those women who carry pitchers on their heads and the meditating Buddhist monks. Most of the photographs I studied for what I would now call visual feedback seemed to be of Japanese Zen monks – perhaps not surprisingly from the land of the Nikon, Pentax, Olympus, and so on.

Everybody I knew agreed that those women with pitchers on their heads were models of graceful and poised posture. It seemed to me that fundamental to their good posture was the upward energy that went into carrying an object on the head. My own experiments indicated that this upward energy was not a thrusting but an inner direction and awareness. The neck did not need to be tensed with a light to moderate weight on the head and the upper body felt uplifted and buoyant. At the same time the lower body would need to be firmly 'earthed' with good support from the lower abdomen and the weight evenly distributed over the two legs and feet.

What I am saying, of course, is that I was independently arriving at truths about poised posture that were given expression in manuals on Zen and also, it turned out eventually, in books on Alexander's postural training.

My belief that the Alexander method could be written about in a straightforward and practical manner was rewarded in 1978 by the appearance of not just one but two books of simple and direct instruction, both written by women. One appeared in America and one in Britain. The American book was *The Alexander Technique: The Revolutionary Way to Use Your Body for Total Energy*, by Sarah Barker. The British publication was *Stand Straight Without Strain: The Original Exercises of F. Matthias Alexander*, by Marie Beuzeville Byles.

Marie Byles writes: 'His (Alexander's) technique, mental, physical, and relaxational, is extremely simple and why the practical side has never been written down is hard to understand.'

In fact, a clear and practical book about the Alexander method published in London five years before the two books I have mentioned was Jack Vinten Fenton's *Choice of Habit*, which has the subtitle 'Poise, Free Movement and the Practical Use of the Body'. This book concentrates on work in postural training with schoolchildren, as I described earlier, and the photographs illustrating good and bad posture are of schoolchildren. I did not come across a copy of the book until after reading the books by Sarah Barker and Marie Byles. Reading Mr Fenton's book then gave me the opportunity to see how well he had used the Alexander method with schoolchildren.

Cultivating good posture in schoolchildren should begin at an early age. Professor John Dewey (1859–1952), the eminent American philosopher, psychologist and educationist, wrote of the Alexander technique:

But the method is not one of remedy; it is one of constructive education. Its proper field of application is with the young, with the growing generation, in order that they may come to possess as early as possible in life a correct standard of sensory appreciation and self-judgement. When once a reasonably adequate part of a new generation has become properly coordinated, we shall have assurance for the first time that men and women in the future will be able to stand on their own feet, equipped with satisfactory psychophysical equilibrium, to meet with readiness, confidence and happiness instead of with fear, confusion and discontent, the buffetings and contingencies of their surroundings.

What is involved is training of the kinaesthetic or 'body motion feeling' sense, which has become faulty in many people. One learns through doing, a principle of education that Professor Dewey strongly advocated.

'Use' is a key concept in the Alexander method. Sarah Barker sums it up: 'Good use means moving the body with maximum balance and coordination of all parts so that only the effort absolutely needed is expended.' I call this poised movement. She also neatly sums up the basic movement on which everything else depends in the method. 'As you begin any movement or act, move your whole head upward and away from your whole body, and let your whole body lengthen by following that upward direction.'

This is an easing up, not a thrusting up. The direction upward should be taken to mean easing the head away from the pelvis, the body following, which may on some occasions mean moving the head and trunk in a diagonal, horizontal or downward movement. Head, neck and back stay in alignment as much as possible, which means most of the time.

With this easing up – not an effort but a thought or visualized idea – the spine is freed from compression and the head does not go back to initiate a movement, as Alexander had found himself doing.

The benefit of this basic control is tested by using it in sitting down on a chair and standing up. Use an ordinary table chair so that you can keep your back straight. Keep your feet flat on the floor and a little apart. Lean forward so that head, neck and back stay in alignment by letting your head move upwards and your body following and lengthening without a break. The head leads; it is not pushed up from below by the body. The now upwards and diagonal movement of the head continues and takes you on to your feet in a standing position. To sit down, you again tilt head, neck and back forward slightly and lower your bottom on to the chair while thinking of the body lengthening, thus avoiding moving the head back and compressing the spine.

People who compress the spine in making movements subject the spine and the nervous system to damaging wear and tear, for they are doing it millions of times.

It is claimed that the Alexander method greatly benefits health. Dr Wilfrid Barlow, a teacher of the method, says that users of the Alexander principle – 'use affects functioning' – 'appear to live longer and more healthily'. He based this claim on an investigation of the lives of men and women who had been taught Alexander's postural training.

The primary control is the key to the method, and training consists of consciously using it for some time when initiating an action. Word formulas are used, much in the manner of those given earlier for use in autogenic training. The precise wording may differ slightly according to which Alexander instructor is listened to. For Sarah Barker the key phrasing is *head moving delicately upward, letting body follow*. Alexander's instruction *head forward and up* must have caused many of his readers receiving no practical instruction in the method to behave like a man with a tight collar stud and thrust the jaw forward and up. With only this word formula and little more to make a judgement on, it was hardly surprising that H. G. Wells mocked George Bernard Shaw and other users of the Alexander method as 'swan neckers'.

It is essential to realize that the primary control counters the tendency of the great majority of people, in the West at any rate, to accompany actions by tilting the head back, shortening and contracting the neck and pressing the head down on the top of the spine where the top vertebra (atlas vertebra) joins the occipital bone at the base of the skull. So the thought *head forward and up* really means *tilt forward* and not thrusting it forward, a postural habit one sees in photographs and films of both Hitler and Mussolini.

Alexander observed that when most people sat down on a chair or got up from it, they threw back their head, stiffening and shortening the neck muscles and compressing the spine. Dr Wilfrid Barlow became a teacher of the Alexander method in 1940, just after the outbreak of war, and had the opportunity to study the body use of 105 young soldiers between the ages of seventeen and twenty-two. He fixed a tapemeasure to the backs of their heads and made an ink mark over the prominent vertebra where the neck joins the chest at the back: if you reach up the spine with one hand you can feel it on yourself. The soldiers were then asked to sit down. Only one of the 105 young men did not pull back his head and so move the tape downwards as he sat down. Fifty-six moved it down two inches or more, forty-three between one and two inches. The youngest men, significantly, tended to have less head movement than the slightly older ones. If we observe young children we see natural easy body use, but as they progress to the sedentary life of the classroom postural faults appear, including head and neck contraction.

To return again to a satisfactory phrase for the primary control or basic movement, Dr Barlow gives *head forward and up, back lengthen and widen*. Remember that head forward is tilt forward from the ears, chin staying level. The addition of *back lengthen and widen* is helpful. Alexander included exercises in expanding the lower ribcage, so that his male trainees found they had after some months to order a new size of waistcoat.

Sarah Barker's formula has the merit of being easily understood and carried out. It helps to think of the head as a kind of block unit in thinking of the upward direction, upward meaning away from the body and not always vertical direction. Dr Barlow adds back lengthening and widening. Marie Byles, I find, brings it all together to provide a useful body image:

*Let the neck be free*
*Let the head be tilted forward and up*
*Chin in*
*To let the back lengthen and widen*

My only reservation about Marie Byle's formula is that some people might pull in the chin too strongly and contract the muscles at the back of the neck. My own experience is that if the neck is relaxed and the head tilted forward and up the chin takes the right position naturally.

My own choice of formula brings together elements from those of Alexander, Barlow, Barker and Byles.

*Neck relaxed and free*
*Head tilted forward*
*Head easing up*
*Back easing up and widening*

I have taken some time with the primary movement because it is the key to success with the Alexander method. It should be applied consciously on numerous occasions in a variety of activities. Try it going up a flight of stairs or steps and note the way the lead with the head 'floats' you up. Remember that when the body follows the head, the neck is relaxed and head, neck and back stay in alignment.

Poor body use, once habitual, can be difficult to overcome. Alexander taught a principle that Aldous Huxley and others thought important: that wrong body use can be inhibited by the rational mind if means rather than ends are thought of. The stages of the formula for the primary control are means; thinking of the end goal of rising from a chair without throwing back the head would be thinking of the end. By focusing attention on the means the end comes of its own accord. There could be valuable lessons here for physical education in schools and elsewhere.

Alexander believed in rational conscious control. Marie Byles prefers the word 'relaxation' to 'inhibition', and sees the

Alexander method as surrender to the life force, to 'It', to a Taoist-like trust in the natural order. She experiences no difficulty in combining Eastern attitudes with the Alexander principle.

## THE ALEXANDER METHOD AND HARA

I have myself experienced no difficulty in combining the Oriental poised posture, including the concept of hara, with Alexander's postural training. Photographs of poised Orientals and of people who have been trained in the Alexander method show similar alignment of head, neck and back. And accounts of Japanese postural training contain material that links up with descriptions of the Alexander method. My own experience confirms that the two can work together. A working synthesis of Eastern and Western techniques of poised living is fruitful at various levels and in various combinations.

The upward direction of the head and body is repeatedly referred to in manuals on Zen by Japanese teachers. A frequent image is that of a string attached to the hairs on top of one's head being gently pulled as though by a puppeteer. Sometimes the trainee is instructed to grasp some hairs on the top back of the head and pull upwards, an exercise given by Marie Byles in her book on the Alexander method as being one of 'the original exercises of F. Matthias Alexander'. A breathing exercise she gives – a whispered 'Ah!' – appears in Zen and Indian Yoga instruction, and one or two more of Alexander's exercises will not be unfamiliar to students of Yoga and Zen. This out of ten exercises.

Karlfried Von Durckheim says that once the body's centre of gravity is found – hara, or more precisely the tanden – the whole upper body feels free, and the personality with it. The spinal column feels as though it is being pushed up from below. He contrasts right posture with wrong posture in which the shoulders are forced back, the chest thrust out and the belly and lower back drawn in, cramping the vital centre in the middle body. In wrong posture, too, the head is bent backwards so that

the skull crushes down on the top of the spine, compressin~~~~~
along its full length. In right posture the body is naturally held
erect and the head, neck and spine ease upward without any
striving on the part of the will. 'The difference in the tension of
the neck is a special criterion of right posture,' says Karl Von
Durckheim. 'It is as if a secret power soared up lightly from
below and culminated in the free carriage of the head.' These
words about posture in hara could come from any manual on
the Alexander method.

Standing upright is a good test of applying the balance of
tension and relaxation that is applied relaxation, that is, poise. If
you relaxed fully you would crumple to the floor. For the
novice, the 'vital centre' is easier to sense in a sitting rather than
in a standing position. But stand with feet a little apart, bodyweight evenly distributed over both legs and feet, apply the
Alexander formula, and see *what* happens.

*Neck relaxed and free*
*Head tilted forward*
*Head easing up*
*Back easing up and widening*

Silently think the words and accompany them with an inwardly
visualized body image. When experienced, the formula can be
reduced to *neck – head – back*. Attend to the means whereby
poised posture is achieved. Let it happen.

Now how do you feel? How especially do you feel in the
abdomen below the navel. You should find that the upper body
is buoyant and that you feel taller, your centre of gravity has
shifted downwards, and the lower abdomen has acquired firmness and strength. The adjustment is slight but there is a
considerable transformation in body management and in how
you feel. If your neck is relaxed and free, you can turn your
head from side to side without experiencing the grating sensations which one gets if the head is pressing down on the top
vertebra.

Western and Eastern techniques of poise can be integrated

and each contributes something to the other method as well as to the combined result.

## EXERCISES

1. The human head is very heavy for its size. A baby's head has to be supported until the neck muscles are strong enough to hold the weighty head upright. The baby achieves this strengthening by repeatedly raising his or her head from the cot or pram and holding it in a vertical position for several seconds. Usually the knees are drawn up.

Adults whose posture has become faulty should be willing to make use of any helpful exercises and to imitate the baby if necessary. Lie flat on your back on a rug or blanket on the floor. Raise your knees and keep your lower back and shoulders flat on the floor. It may take some practice before the lower back settles down, but you should be able to keep the shoulders right down. Take a breath. Breathing out, raise your head to vertical. Keep the head up five to ten seconds before lowering the back of the head to the floor. Repeat five times. Then stand up slowly and note the new feeling in the head, neck and upper body. Acquiring improved body feeling is important, as we saw in training for muscular relaxation.

2. A lot can be learned about your posture by standing with your back to a wall but with your heels about two inches from it and your feet about eighteen inches apart. Stand in your best erect posture, then slowly sway your body back to the wall without moving your feet. Your shoulderblades and your buttocks should make contact with the wall simultaneously. Both sides of the body should also make contact simultaneously; if your posture is slightly twisted, one shoulderblade and/or buttock will make contact with the wall a fraction of a second before the other side. If your shoulders make contact before your buttocks, you are carrying your pelvis too far forward. If your buttocks hit the wall before your shoulderblades, you are carrying your pelvis too far back. If the back of

your skull is firm against the wall, you are retracting the he. another postural fault. On discovery of the above postural fault. through this test, the necessary adjustments may be made. Note how the new position feels, then walk away from the wall while retaining the new posture. It may not last, but you are getting the feeling of right posture.

There remains the commonest fault uncovered by the preceding test: an exaggerated curve in the lower back, the lumbar region. Most books about posture advise standing against a wall and trying to flatten the lower back against the wall. This exercise can be aided in several ways.

Now you can move your heels in against the wall, together with shoulderblades and buttocks. If there is no contact between your lower back and the wall, bend your knees forward, and flex your pelvis by lowering your buttocks and tipping your sexual parts more towards the front. This brings your lower back in contact with the wall. It is a useful exercise to slide your lower back down the wall several times.

Another way to 'flatten' the lumbar region against the wall is to raise both arms forward to the horizontal position. Do this five times to become familiar with the feeling.

Yet another aid to reducing the curve in the lower back is to drop your shoulders and rise on your toes. Rise on your toes five times while focusing your attention on the lower back.

Conclude each exercise by walking away from the wall while retaining the corrected posture.

3. Lie on your back on the floor and draw your feet back some way towards your buttocks. Take a breath. Breathing out, raise the lower bones of your spine off the floor, pressing down with the soles of your feet. Only these 'tail' bones (the coccyx) should be lifted, for the idea again is to flatten the full length of the back against the floor.

4. Teachers of the Alexander method gently ease up the occipital bone at the base of the skulls of their clients. You can do it yourself. Place the palms of your hands at the sides of your

neck, fingers meeting at the back of the neck. Raise the fingers and ease up the occipital bone for about five seconds. Apply gentle pressure upwards on the bone five times.

The purpose behind this exercise is to help the head take and give you the feeling of the correct position in relation to the neck and spine.

5. On performing the preceding exercise in which the occipital bone is pressed upwards, you will feel that the back of the top of your head is the highest point in your erect posture. A further exercise to help the head tilt forward and up is to grasp a few hairs on the top back of the head and tug them gently upwards for a few seconds. Do this five times. Alexander used to say that he 'hung himself' every night before getting into bed.

In performing exercises 4 and 5 you should think of the primary control and its formula and have a sensed inner picture of the poised alignment of head, neck and spine. It also helps to have an inner image of the movements of the head. The skull rocks forwards and backwards on the vertebral axis by means of a pair of joints formed by projections of the occipital bone and sockets in the first cervical or neck vertebra, called the atlas. When the head is turned from side to side, the skull and the atlas move together on a toothlike projection of the second cervical vertebra, called the axis. This movement should be easy and devoid of gritty sensations.

## HOLDING THE PATTERN IN EVERYDAY ACTIVITIES

This is really the most important set of exercises. Poised posture should not be reserved for meditation or special exercise periods, but should be applied in life's everyday situations.

The alignment and pattern of good use of the head, neck and spine means that you bend from the pelvis keeping the upper body in line to get up from a chair or to jack-knife and sit down on one. You do the same when bending forward to pick something up from a table or desk. If the object you wish to pick up is on the floor, then you bend your knees and squat down as a young child will be seen to do, again holding the upper body pattern.

Good body use saves energy and prevents wear and tear on the spine, joints, ligaments and muscles, as well as protecting against injury. Good patterns should be maintained in play as well as in work. Poised posture is the hallmark of the skilled athlete, just as it is of the brilliant instrumentalist or dancer.

In walking, jogging or running remember that the head should not go back to compress the spine, a move likely soon to produce spinal trouble and back pains. Lead with the head, body following, and grace and ease in motion will result.

Of home and class exercise systems, Hatha Yoga with its variety of postures (*asanas*) is conducive to improved posture; on the other hand, learning good body use as discussed in this chapter means you can bring more to, and get more from your Yoga exercises.

The slow motion graceful movements of the Chinese exercise system *Tai chi ch'uan* benefit posture, and the remarks I have just made about Yoga apply to these exercises also. Unfortunately, it is difficult to learn the movements from reading books, however profusely illustrated. Yoga exercises can be learned from books, being static postures and not movement exercises.

## SUPINE ABDOMINAL BREATHING

This chapter has concentrated more on posture than on breathing because once poised posture is established, poised breathing follows naturally.

Shallow high upper-chest breathing goes with slumped and rigid postures, in both of which the muscles of respiration are impeded from carrying out their full action of expansion and contraction. In poised posture the respiratory muscles are set free and function harmoniously. You will benefit from having an image of this healthful action, and from your kinaesthetic sense recording the feeling.

In poised breathing upper, middle and lower lungs take in

and release air; and all of the respiratory muscles participate fully. The largest of these muscles is the diaphragm, below your chest, which acts like a piston, flattening out and moving down on breathing in and rising and regaining its dome shape on breathing out. The abdominal wall responds to the pistonlike action of the powerful diaphragm muscle – Enrico Caruso could push a grand piano across a room with his – by swelling out on inhalation of air and falling back on exhalation of air.

The exercise of supine abdominal feeling is an effective way to become familiar with the feeling of diaphragmatic and abdominal breathing. It is the most healthful and relaxed way to breathe, worth memorizing and acquiring as a habit for use throughout life. Abdominal breathing can also play a useful part in practising meditation.

Lie flat on your back, your legs extended though not 'locked' at the knees, your arms bent and the palms of your hands resting on your abdomen so that the tips of your longest fingers meet just over the navel. The backs of your upper arms rest on the floor, while your forearms are held in against your ribs. In this relaxed position the action of the breathing muscles can be easily experienced. These muscles belong to the thoracic cage, the diaphragm and the abdomen. All other muscles should be relaxed and unobtrusive. A minimum of loose clothing should be worn.

If you are able to let the lower back flatten and make contact with the floor, a sign of advanced skill in posture, the action of the thoracic cage will be more strongly sensed.

Before giving your full attention to your breathing, make your final adjustments to your posture while lying perfectly still. For poised breathing we need poised posture, whether standing, sitting or, as now, lying down. So go over the formula and let relaxation and poise happen.

*Neck relaxed and free*
*Head tilted forward*
*Head easing up*
*Back easing up and widening*

The head and spine will, of course, be here easing in a direction away from the pelvis. The whole body will feel as though it is lengthening. You are now ready for poised breathing and for awareness of it.

Take a slow deep breath to a point short of cramming or discomfort. Be fully mindful of the muscle movements entailed: the expansion of the ribs against the forearms, the diaphragm flattening out and moving down under your hands to swell out the belly and raise your hands.

Pause for a second or two and then let the air slowly flow out of your lungs and note the reverse muscular process taking place. The ribs fall in, the diaphragm rises and the abdomen falls back and flattens beneath the palms of your hands.

Perform two more of these slow controlled breaths, then spend three to five minutes relaxing and breathing naturally. *It* breathes. Let it happen. But be aware all the time of it happening so that you will remember what it feels like.

Practise this poised breathing in a supine position once or twice daily for a week. Continue it for a second week, but add a similar period of awareness of breathing practice while sitting upright. On a third week of practice be aware of relaxed breathing while supine, sitting erect and standing upright. By then you should know what poised breathing is about and be establishing it as a habit accompanied by poised posture.

Your short period of training in awareness of breathing will prove useful for success in our next deep relaxation method – meditation.

# 8 Meditation for All

## THE IRON BIRD FLIES TO THE WEST

In many thousands of homes in the USA and in Europe something strange is happening: mothers, fathers, daughters and sons are sitting quietly for fifteen to twenty minutes twice a day and meditating in the manner of Indian Yogins or Far Eastern Buddhists. They may not always be doing it for the same reasons as the Yogins or Buddhists, but they are practising basic techniques from the age-old spiritual disciplines of Eastern mystical religions.

On 24 May 1972, the House of Representatives of the State of Illinois passed House Resolution No. 677. The gist of it may be gathered from the following extracts:

*Whereas*, Transcendental Meditation is a simple natural technique of gaining deep rest and relaxation which is easily learned by everyone; and

*Whereas*, School officials have noted a lessening of student unrest and an improvement in grades and student-parent-teacher relationships among practitioners of Transcendental Meditation, and

*Whereas*, Physiological experiments provide evidence that through the regular practice of TM (twice daily for 15–20 minutes) the main causes of hypertension, anxiety, high blood pressure, cardiac arrest, and other psychosomatic illnesses are removed; and . . .

*Resolved*, By the House of Representatives of the Seventy-seventh General Assembly of the State of Illinois, that all educational institutions, especially those under State of Illinois jurisdiction, be strongly encouraged to study the feasibility of courses in Transcendental Meditation and the Science of Creative Intelligence (SCI) on their campuses and in their facilities, . . . etc., etc.

Interest in Eastern meditation developed in the 1960s in the United States, mainly among young people interested in altered states of consciousness. By the early seventies the practice of meditation had lost its 'exotic' image and was being practised by people of all ages, social classes and educational backgrounds. The State of Illinois was able to encourage the teaching of meditation in their educational institutions.

The sponsor of the resolution was Representative Willard ('Bingo Bill') Murphy, a politician of the old school and not the type of man to be associated with anything too 'way out' or lacking in practical worth. He pointed out that he had started meditating to set a good example to his sons at a time when many young people were taking to drugs for 'highs'. He had suffered from frequent headaches, but after starting meditating he had not had a headache in three years. He reported, too, that meditation had made his mind clearer, and had made him a more alert and a more tolerant driver.

Transcendental meditation has become the form of meditation most widely practised in the West. Its promotion has been based chiefly on its relaxation value, but the technique belongs to Hindu Yoga. There are many thousands of Western practitioners of Buddhist meditation – Theravadan, Tibetan and Zen. The publication of books on Yoga, Buddhism, Tantra, and Sufism has grown greatly.

There is an Indian saying that when the iron bird flies in the sky then the mystical teaching based on meditation will go to the West. Well, it has happened.

## WHAT KIND OF MEDITATION?

The meditation that we are interested in is not the intellectual exercise that most dictionaries continue to say it is. On the contrary, it is the use of psychological devices to reduce thought and to treat those images and thoughts that do come unbidden into the mind with passive indifference. They are ignore or watched in a detached, disinterested manner.

The methods used in most forms of Eastern meditation quieten and relax the mind. They are based on bare attention, in which there is no intellectual comment or judgement. You sit in poised posture, breathe quietly and smoothly, and let passive attention dwell on a meditation object. You let meditation happen.

The basic technique of a meditation used in the mystical psychologies of the East can be practised either with or without religious, metaphysical or philosophical associations. Dr Herbert Benson of the Harvard Medical School studied meditation methods and worked out the bare essentials of the practice for use by patients who would benefit from body–mind relaxation.

Mystical enlightenment or higher consciousness is the *raison d'être* of meditation, but Dr Benson was interested in the elements in meditation practice that elicited the relaxation response, the opposite of the fight or flight response that explained stress reactions. He had already discovered through laboratory testing of meditators that meditation decreased breathing rate, oxygen consumption, heart rate and blood lactate to levels not found outside very deep sleep or hibernation.

Dr Benson found that the integrated relaxation response could be elicited by traditional methods of meditation as long as they contained four basic elements. These are:

1 A quiet environment
2 A comfortable posture, usually sitting so as to prevent sleep or heavy drowsiness
3 An object for the attention to dwell on (a meditation object)
4 Passive awareness

A passive attitude is the most important component. I will be showing later how it can be used at any time for bare attention to what is happening at the moment. But in this chapter we are concerned with how to meditate intensively in periods of sitting motionless in poised posture. Such formal meditation practice gets maximum results in inducing psychophysical relaxation and in establishing meditation consciousness. With regular daily practice, both the relaxation and the awareness may be carried into activity and consciousness at other times of the day.

Practise meditation for about twenty minutes once or twice a day. If only meditating once a day, you should practise progressive relaxation, autogenic training, self-hypnosis, a biofeedback relaxation for twenty minutes at another time in the day. For best results from practice, let six hours or more separate two sessions of relaxation.

## SIMPLE EFFECTIVE TECHNIQUES

The techniques of meditation now practised within or outside the major religions mostly originated as methods of spiritual training, principally as ways of transcending the striving, restless ego and penetrating to pure consciousness.

Basically, the techniques are simple when stripped of their doctrinal wrappings. You become aware of your breathing, you repeat a word or a sound inwardly, you look at something steadily or visualize something in your mind, you listen steadily to a sound, or you sustain loving attention in your heart. Attention is the heart of meditation. Any of your senses may be used for sustained awareness.

The techniques given here have been chosen for their simplicity and for their emotional and intellectual neutrality. They are easy to learn, of a kind that can be practised by every reader and they rapidly induce the relaxation response.

Let us look at the four essential elements of meditation again, this time in more detail. Various points will be made that the newcomer to meditation should remember. However, thinking about how to meditate during meditation is no longer

...editation. The time to think about the technique of meditation is beforehand. Then sit down in poised posture, close your eyes and just meditate.

Three essentials for effective meditation are poised posture, poised breathing and poised awareness. Poised breathing occurs if you sit in poised posture and relax, and if your habitual breathing is healthfully based on using the abdomen as well as the diaphragm and the intercostal muscles between the ribs. We will therefore give most attention to poised posture and poised awareness. But first, some practical considerations.

## CONDITIONS FOR MEDITATION

The beginner in meditation especially needs conditions in which environmental stimuli are as low as possible. Experienced meditators may be able to relax and turn their attention inwards in circumstances that beginners would find distracting. This is a useful ability, just as it is to learn to attain muscular relaxation in a situation of some discomfort.

Closing the eyes cuts down instantly on a considerable source of stimuli. Poised posture and poised breathing also keep down stimuli, the former through staying motionless and having low muscle tonus, the latter through gentle rhythmical breathing.

Wash your hands and face at least before meditating. Brush your teeth and rinse out your mouth with fresh water. Splash your eyes with cold water. Your stomach should feel neither full nor empty. Empty your bladder, and your bowel too, if possible.

Wear the minimum of loose clothing that circumstances and room temperature allow. Take off your shoes.

Unless your nostrils are blocked, breathe through them. Keep your lips lightly together but your teeth slightly parted. Let your tongue lie flat and relaxed in your mouth with its tip against your lower teeth.

## POISED POSTURE

The ability to relax specific muscles and keep muscular tension to a minimum will prove helpful in settling quickly into useful states of awareness during meditation. In most meditative traditions the posture you adopt for sitting is considered significant. Thus the methods of postural adjustment given in the preceding chapter will be found relevant to establishing good meditation posture.

In sitting for meditation the body is kept perfectly still and in a state of perfect balance and equilibrium.

Sitting motionless for fifteen to twenty minutes is itself a considerable relaxation benefit for Westerners brought up in societies obsessed with 'getting things done', 'getting on', 'go getting', and so on. For many Westerners sitting still for even five minutes is an achievement. If you do not sit still there is little chance of your mind finding the calm, clear awareness that is the essence of the meditative experience. Movement is distraction. Hence the need for a stable, well-balanced sitting posture for meditation.

In the Zen schools poised posture is considered to be essential for zazen or sitting meditation. The Zen masters teach that body and mind are one and that the body parts should be arranged harmoniously, with the centre of gravity just below the navel, if the mind is to find its own poise. Regulation of the body and its breathing are the foundation for regulation of the mind. Bodily stability and mental stability go together.

Dr Tomio Hirai, who has spent many years studying the psychology and physiology of Zen meditation, says 'the mentally stable person can remain physically stable for a fixed period of time. The smaller the range of his body movements in that period of time, the more stable his mind is likely to be.' One of his studies was into the movements and non-movement of three groups of people. A group of Zen priests, of 'ordinary' people, and of neurotic patients meditated while sitting in various positions. In every position there were barely any movements from the Zen priests, considerably more movement from the 'ordinary' group, and much erratic movement from the neurotic people.

Dr Hirai reported that although the Zen meditator sits very still and appears static 'he is actually filled with abundant vitality'. He also found that the traditional sitting postures 'do not apply undue pressure on the vertebrae and therefore do not constrict or dull the autonomous nerves in the vicinity of the vertebrae.'

Dr Hirai also found that the Zen priests' sleeping postures continued the principles of their meditation postures. They slept on their sides, with their spines comfortably straight and heads and spines in line. Again there was no pressure on the spinal nerves. He concluded that the sleeping Zen posture was favourable to healthy working of the autonomic nervous system, which controls the heart, legs, stomach and other internal organs.

Another interesting fact from the same investigation is that measurement of the brain waves of sleeping Zen priests revealed that even in deepest sleep, with the EEG showing the very slow theta and delta waves, the Zen priests were always ready to respond to outside stimuli.

## SITTING POSTURES FOR MEDITATION

*Sitting in a straight-backed chair*. Keep your legs a little apart and your feet firmly on the floor. Have a cushion between your lower back and the back of the chair. Torso and thighs should form a rightangle and also upper and lower legs. All the advice about poised posture given in the preceding chapter should be applied in the sitting postures for meditation. Find the point of balance on the sitting bone and keep head, neck and back comfortably straight. Think upwards with your head. The feeling is of firm balance and poise. The abdomen is relaxed so that deep, restful breathing ensues spontaneously. Rest the back of your left hand in the palm of your right hand and hold your hands horizontally against your lower belly, your wrists supported by your upper thighs where they reach the hip joints. Reverse hand positions if you are left-handed.

The combination of relaxation and alertness would not be possible sinking into and lying back in an armchair.

*The traditional crosslegged postures.* Though meditation may be practised sitting in a chair, the traditional Eastern meditation postures have special value and if you can sit comfortably in any of them you should do so. You may wish to sit in a chair for a few weeks for meditation, while becoming used to the crosslegged or other traditional sitting posture by using them for a few minutes at a time at intervals during the day. If you sit in them for short periods to read, watch television, listen to radio or records, and so on, you will find that your leg and hip joints will become progressively more flexible. In a few weeks you will probably be able to start meditating while sitting on the floor in the Eastern manner.

Sit on a thick firm cushion and have a thinner cushion or rug below your knees to prevent distracting discomfort. Sitting on a cushion makes these traditional sitting postures much easier to achieve with both knees down as they should be.

The full *lotus posture* is the most difficult for Westerners, though some manage it quite quickly. You pick up your right foot and place it high up on your left thigh and pick up your left foot and place it high up on your right thigh, or in reverse sequence. The soles of the feet should be turned up. The higher you place your feet on the thighs the more easy it is to lower your knees to the floor.

In the *half-lotus posture* only one foot is upturned on a thigh. The heel of the other is drawn in against the pubic bone, pulling the foot high up the thigh so as to lower the knee to the floor.

To sit in *easy yoga posture*, simply cross your ankles and keep your knees down as far as possible. They will lower to the floor with practice. You should then sit in one of the other traditional postures, which provide greater stability.

In *perfect yoga posture* you fully flex one leg and draw the heel in against the perineum (between genitals and anus). The other leg is flexed and the sole of the foot upturned and tucked into the groove between the calf and thigh of the other leg. Both knees should be on the floor.

*Burmese posture*. This is highly recommended when the above crosslegged positions cause discomfort before the end of the fifteen to twenty minutes given to meditation. Description of it is unaccountably missing in the various manuals of meditation, with the exception of Philip Kapleau's *The Three Pillars of Zen*, where it is described and illustrated. Yet people can often be seen sitting in this stable but comfortable position in photographs of group meditation in the East. See, for example, photographs which appear in Shindai Sekiguchi's *Zen: A Manual for Westerners*. I hit on this sitting posture for my own use some years before coming across it in Philip Kapleau's book.

In Burmese posture – Philip Kapleau modifies with the words 'so-called' – the legs are not actually crossed. One leg is fully flexed with the heel drawn in against the perineum. The other leg is then flexed and the foot drawn back to rest on the floor in front of the other foot or ankle.

In all the above postures beginners find they need to thrust out their buttocks slightly to centre on the sitting bone. You should be able to sway forwards and backwards easily like one of those little wooden figures with a rounded and weighted bottom that come upright when pushed in any direction. Also make a few circling motions with your poised upper body, moving from the hips, clockwise and anticlockwise. The centre of gravity should be just below the navel. Relax the belly so that you breathe easily and deeply.

The combination of Eastern hara and Western Alexander method described in the preceding chapter applies here again. Think of leading upwards with the head, following with the torso from the firm base of the lower belly. Shindai Sekiguchi writes: 'While keeping your knees down, stretch your spine upward and straight as though you were trying to push your head through the ceiling.' He also suggests, again in accord with Alexander, that the meditator should imagine a thread attached to the hairs on top of his or her head which are being pulled upwards.

I would add a reminder to the reader that stretching upwards need only be a very small, but important, adjustment. Any of the verbal formulas of the Alexander method given in the preceding chapter will be found suitable for a meditation posture.

Nose and navel should be in perpendicular line. You may find it helpful to sit in front of a mirror against whose glass a piece of string has been blue-tacked as a postural plumbline.

The hand positions suggested for sitting in a chair apply in all positions. The dominant hand is usually 'immobilized' by being kept below the other hand. In the lotus postures the hands may rest on the heels or one heel for the half-lotus. Zen meditators are taught to bring their thumb tips together, but any comfortable position for the thumb will be satisfactory.

The postural poise established in meditation and the inner posture that goes with it should be carried into daily life, whatever activity you are engaged in.

## CLOSE YOUR EYES

Japanese Zen meditators keep their eyes half open and gaze at a point on the floor a few feet in front of them. But in most other traditions of meditation the eyes are kept closed to help the attention turn inwards. The eyes are kept open in Zen meditation to ward off sleep, but most meditators who close their eyes find they do not go to sleep unless very tired, when sleep should be accepted with as little fuss as thoughts and images appearing in the mind. Alpha wave production in the brain, which is associated with mental relaxation, occurs most easily when the eyes are closed, though it also occurs in experienced meditators who have their eyes open.

## POISED BREATHING

Having settled in poised sitting posture, like a pendulum that has come to rest after some gentle rocking movements, become aware of your breathing. Take three slow deep breaths down into the relaxed abdomen, tightening the lower belly slightly on each exhalation. This helps establish the centre of gravity in the lower belly and encourages slow deep breathing. Thereafter the breath need not be controlled, but left to find its own easy, slow rhythm as meditation and relaxation deepen.

You have now taken a posture and a way of breathing that reduces body and breathing sensation to a minimum and so promotes poised attention.

## POISED AWARENESS

The Zen master Ikkyu was asked to write some wisdom maxims. He dipped his brush in ink and wrote a single word – 'Attention'. Asked to add something more, Ikkyu wrote: 'Attention. Attention.' And when the questioner complained that he could see nothing profound in what the Zen master had written, Ikkyu then wrote: 'Attention. Attention. Attention.'

Meditation is bare attention or passive awareness, whether in formal sitting meditation or during some everyday activity. If you think of meditation as awareness then you give it reality. There is nothing strange or exotic about it. The awareness of sitting meditation is that of the boy or girl you once were sitting still and listening to the sound of the rain or watching the silent fall of snow. It is the awareness of the fisherman watching his float and of the man or woman who gazes at his or her reflection in a mirror casually without commenting thought or aroused feelings. It is 'just looking', 'just listening', or 'just being aware'.

The travelling sage J. Krishnamurti says that meditation is 'the experiencing of what is without naming'. Discriminative thought is missing; there is only bare attention. We are more familiar with this special quality of poised awareness in childhood than in adult life, which accounts in a major way for the nostalgia of childhood memories. We recall, vividly or vaguely, the periods of bare awareness and of pure being we knew in childhood, before perceptions and experiences lost their freshness and became habituated and automatized.

Meditation has a special quality that comes from attention without thought. The quality becomes purer as meditation deepens. Then come periods between thoughts so pure and free of content that, as one meditator put it, 'You don't know you're there, but you know you've been'. Breathing stops or nearly stops, body and mind are 'dropped' or 'fall off'. This pure awareness is called *samadhi* in Eastern meditation. These are the moments of purest mental relaxation.

Meditation attention, bare because free of thought, relaxed yet alert, I am calling poised awareness. This is a logical further-ance of my calling muscular relaxation plus alertness poised action.

Meditation is freedom from thought. But when thought breaks in, as it certainly will, then continue to be passively aware; make no fuss, show no irritation, no matter how many times awareness of the meditation object or the constant process is interrupted. In meditation, stilling the mind is the aim, but it is not obtained by using will power to suppress images and verbal thinking. They are passively noted and then you return to awareness of the meditation object or process. Thoughts starved of your interest or reaction become fewer and weaker, so that gaps between them become more frequent. Linear, chain-reaction thinking does not develop. Thoughts and images are isolated without their associations and pass across the mind like pale clouds crossing an expanse of blue sky. Bassui, a fourteenth-century Zen master, said that meditation is 'no more than looking into one's own mind, neither despising nor cherishing the thoughts that arise.'

Passive awareness is the key to tranquillity meditation and to eliciting the relaxation response. Maintain detached awareness. Don't start thinking about how you are meditating. Don't anticipate results, which is thinking again. Let your attention dwell on the rise and fall of your abdomen or on the silently repeated word in the techniques that follow, which have been chosen for their neutrality, simplicity and effectiveness. Effortless concentration will develop, but do not force it. Your attention is like a torch beam, and you have only to direct it repeatedly where it is to go. When it wanders, bring it back. Let go. Open up. Let it happen.

We will restrict ourselves here to two techniques that are suitable and effective for all meditators. They elicit the relaxation response and mental calm. They do not depend on religious faith or devotion.

The first method is awareness of breathing, which is taught especially in Buddhist schools of meditation. The other method is inward repetition of word, syllable or sound, which is a technique most associated with Hindu Mantra Yoga and which is the sole method taught under the name transcendental meditation.

Both these meditation methods are quickly learned and give immediate benefits in improved relaxation, health and energy. They may also be effectively combined, the sound being inwardly 'thought' on each exhalation of breath.

I will also describe an advanced technique with relevance to cultivating an attitude of letting go and of opening up to life.

The following chapter will show how meditation may be practised in daily life, developing relaxed detachment and insight.

## AWARENESS OF BREATHING

Considering that breathing is a constant process, it is surprising how rarely we give it our full attention. Most people are only aware of their breathing when something goes wrong with it: when they choke, or cough, or hold it to prevent noxious fumes or water entering their lungs.

Our breathing is a highly appropriate process on which to focus meditation awareness for several reasons. One is the practical advantage that it is with us all the time, from birth to the moment of death. We can use breathing as a meditation object or process at any time. There is the fact, too, that breathing rhythms are a measure of relaxation and tranquillity. As meditation and relaxation deepen, the breathing becomes slower and smoother. In the moments when thought ceases the breathing also becomes still or barely perceptible. When we are agitated our breathing becomes quick and jerky; when we are tranquil our breathing reflects the mental calm. Some people, too, will be conscious that the Latin *spiritus* means both 'spirit' and 'breath'.

Be aware of air coming into the body and going out. Note the effortlessness of the process if you do not interfere. Air seems to fall in and out. Observe your breathing and let it happen. If you let it flow naturally, your breathing will become very quiet, though you may occasionally take one large breath that you let out like a long sigh. This is due to the great reduction in air intake and oxygen consumption that accompanies meditation; occasionally the body may decide to take in a little more air.

Breathing is an involuntary process, with some voluntary control. Meditation on breathing is useful training in identifying with the Tao or natural flow of nature. In this meditation the ego lets go, loses its hard shell, and one feels as though 'being breathed', though a further stage is simply the feeling of 'just breathing'. First, 'I breathe', then 'I am breathed', then 'breathing' – the experience and nothing more.

Give yourself a focus of awareness. This can be the lower abdomen which, if you are breathing correctly, will swell on each in breath and draw in on each out breath. If your bare attention dwells on the movement of the lower abdomen thought will be reduced and you will experience periods of clear consciousness. When thoughts do occur, either as self-talk in your head or as floating images, view them passively and detachedly. Each time you become aware that your attention has strayed, bring it gently back to awareness of your abdomen about two inches below the navel, the tanden or vital centre. Even if you do not attach the importance to this spot that the Japanese do, it will be a suitable focus of awareness for this meditation. In some Buddhist schools another focus of awareness is given: the place in the nostrils where the air impinges on breathing in and breathing out. Apart from any significance that may be given to the concepts of hara and the tanden, the lower abdomen seems to me to be the focus of awareness most conducive to relaxation and tranquillity. The gentle movement of the abdomen with slow deep breathing is rhythmical and restful and takes awareness well away from the head, which we tend to identify with thought and the ego.

In Buddhist meditation centres the newcomer to meditation is often given a preliminary breathing meditation to that which I have described above. In this other version you count each breath up to ten, and then go back to one again. This may be done on each inhalation and each exhalation: in – one; out – two; and so on – or only on the exhalations. As exhalations are particularly associated with releasing tension, I recommend the latter counting method.

Most beginners in meditation are surprised to find how difficult it can be to keep one's attention on the count to ten; the attention wanders. When this happens and you become aware that it has happened, go back to 'one' again and resume counting breaths. No irritation should be felt. Be tolerant and patient and detached from it all.

The focus of awareness is about two inches below the navel and it helps synchronize the meditation if you think each number as the lower abdomen draws back slightly on each exhalation and, as it were, visually place the number a little below the navel.

This is considered a good beginner's meditation, though one which experienced meditators often like to go back to occasionally. After three or four weeks of counting breaths, drop the counting and see how you get on with simple bare attention of breathing. Counting is a form of mental activity, even if restricted and repetitive, and the less mental activity there is in meditation the better. However, you may feel you would benefit from a few weeks more counting breaths than the three or four I am suggesting; take that course if you wish.

## SAYING THE WORD

This is our second simple meditative technique for eliciting deep relaxation and tranquillity.

As with awareness of breathing or any other meditation method, sit motionless in poised posture in a place where distractions are likely to be few. Breathe through your nostrils and down into your abdomen. Your breathing will become slow, deep and gentle as meditation and relaxation deepen.

You think a word in your head and continue to do so easily and unhurriedly. The process is effortless: there should be no forcing of production of the word or of its retention in the mind. Let it float. If the word vanishes and is replaced by thought or images that arrive uninvited, no matter. Once you become aware that your attention has wandered, introduce the word again. Do this as many times as is necessary during fifteen to twenty minutes' meditation. Relax to the meditation. Let it happen. Sustain passive awareness. The method is simple but effective. Relax and enjoy it.

## WHAT'S THE WORD?

This meditation method occurs in several mystical traditions, but is particularly associated with Hindu Mantra Yoga. A *mantra* is a word, syllable or sound that is repeated aloud or silently as a form of meditation. Hindus attach mystical and occult powers to particular mantras, including all fifty letters of the Sanskrit alphabet. Most mantras have devotional significance – such as the well-known *Om* or *Aum* and *Om mani padme hum*. Many are names of deities.

More than one million Westerners have paid their fees and been initiated into the practice of transcendental meditation (TM), which is the silent mantra. The head of the movement is Maharishi Mahesh Yogi. The method has been updated and presented in a scientific way with emphasis on the way meditation releases stress, but retains the idea of Sanskrit words and syllables having special influences. TM's initiates are said to be given a Sanskrit mantra specially suited to them. In practice many people get the same mantra, including sometimes husbands and wives and friends. Daniel Goleman points out in *The Varieties of the Meditative Experience* that the issue of TM mantras is based on general categories of age, education, and so on. He also points out that though most Westerners are unaware of any meaning in the Sanskrit words, they are known to devotional Hindus. *Shyam* is a name of Lord Krishna and *Aing* is a sound sacred to the Divine Mother.

A train of associations is obviously undesirable, so there are grounds for saying that one should choose a word or sound as meditation object or device that is either meaningless or lacking strong associations. It is not difficult to make up a word that is meaningless, or borrow a foreign word, Sanskrit or otherwise. Zen meditators use the Japanese word *Mu* (*Wu* in Chinese), meaning 'nothing'. I see nothing wrong, however, in making a mantra of a word such as 'peace' that contributes a general ambience of relaxation and tranquillity and does not usually trigger discursive thought. If you were determined to do so, any word can be used as a starting point for thinking; in practice, repetition and familiarity with the mantra prevents its becoming a stimulant of thought.

Dr Herbert Benson, whose study of meditators and meditation methods has already been discussed, has found the inward repetition of a word effective relaxation therapy. He has his patients use the neutral-sounding word 'one'. Its use with a passive attitude elicits the relaxation response.

Early in life the Victorian poet Alfred, Lord Tennyson hit upon the basic technique of Mantra Yoga and of Maharishi Mahesh Yogi's transcendental meditation. He wrote, in a letter, of

a kind of waking trance – this for lack of a better word – I have frequently had, quite up from boyhood, when I have been all alone. This has come upon me through repeating my own name to myself silently, till all at once, as it were out of the intensity of the consciousness of individuality, individuality itself seemed to dissolve and fade away into boundless being, and this is not a confused state but the clearest, the surest of the surest, utterly beyond words – where death was an almost laughable impossibility – the loss of personality (if so it were) seeming no extinction, but the only true life.

Professor John Tyndall wrote that the poet said of his mantra-induced state of mind: 'By God Almighty! there is no delusion in the matter! It is no nebulous ecstasy, but a state of transcendent wonder, associated with absolute clearness of mind.'

Dr Richard Maurice Bucke, a psychiatrist himself familiar with altered states of consciousness, quoted Tennyson's letter in *Cosmic Consciousness* and commented:

Tennyson quite unconsciously was using the means laid down from immemorial time for the attainment of illumination. 'He who thinking of nothing, making the mind cease to work, adhering to uninterrupted meditation, repeating the single syllable OM, meditating on me [Lord Krishna], reached the highest goal' (*Bhagavad Gita*). Of course it makes no differences what word or name is used. What is required is that the action of the mind should be as far as possible suspended, especially that all desires of every kind be stilled, nothing wished or feared, the mind in perfect health and vigour, but held quiescent in a state of calm equipoise.

It would be difficult to better this as an account (published in 1901) of the meditative method and state of awareness – 'the mind in perfect health and vigour, but held quiescent in a state of calm equipoise'. And Dr Bucke's comment, 'of course it makes no difference what word or name is used', was given scientific confirmation by Dr Benson's laboratory studies seventy years later.

## COMBINING METHODS

Dr Herbert Benson has been combining the two simple meditation methods described above with patients at the Beth Israel Hospital of Boston. They become aware of their breathing and then silently say 'one' on each exhalation, continuing the meditation for ten to twenty minutes. He does not specify a localized focus for awareness of breathing. I used this method for some years before reading the *Relaxation Response*, using a different word as mantra. Dr Benson's method closely resembles the Buddhist counting of exhaled breaths, but always staying at 'one'.


## JUST SITTING

This advanced Zen method of meditation, which has the appearance of the utmost simplicity, dispenses with any psychological device to quieten the mind. The meditator 'just sits' in poised posture. I mention it here because it provides useful practice in mindfulness of what is happening here and now, an attitude or inner posture that is valuable for various reasons in active daily life. It acts as a mental hygiene and promotes relaxed and poised living. It will be discussed further in the following chapter.

In the other two methods described there is awareness of breathing and repetition inwardly of a word to bring peace to the mind. In just sitting (*shikan-taza*) the sensations of poised sitting are the nearest one can come to having a constant awareness. There is nothing slack about this meditation. Awareness is passive, yet there is a positive experience of simple being that some people would not hesitate to describe as blissful.

There is no target for effortless concentration. You feel 'open on all sides' – which is the awareness of the perfected Zen swordsman, whose life could be said to depend on his alertness. In shikan-taza you are poised and firmly centred – and brightly aware.

This is the central meditation method of one of the two main schools of Zen – the *Soto* School. The meditation of this school has not received as much publicity in the West as that of the *Rinzai* School. There are several reasons for this. One is that one Japanese Zen writer, D. T. Suzuki, has been so brilliant in writing about Zen for Western readers, and he writes mainly about Rinzai methods. Secondly, the *koan* method of Rinzai practice intrigues Westerners. A koan is a problem that cannot be solved by the intellect. An example: a sound is made by two hands clapping. What sound is made by the clapping of one hand?

That shikan-taza is not minutes of idle reverie may be discerned from its name. *Shikan* means 'nothing but' or 'just', *ta* means 'to hit', and *za* 'to sit'. It has its own sustained mental tonus. You neither strain nor become slack. Remember Bucke's words again: 'the mind in perfect health and vigour, but held quiescent in a state of calm equipoise.' It is the meditative equivalent of riding a bicycle with no hands, but worth practising daily for a few minutes at a separate time from your other meditation practice because mindfulness is useful in everyday living and this purest form of *zazen* develops it.

Readers seeking extended knowledge of meditation methods are referred to my book *Teach Yourself Meditation*.

## WHY MEDITATE?

The main reasons for meditating will already be clear to readers, but will now be brought together.

All the major religions have their systems of meditation. In the Eastern religions, which can also be described as esoteric psychologies, meditation is central in spiritual training, because through its practice the aspirant may come to know his or her real nature and ultimate reality. Christians are no longer so familiar with meditation, as the mystical side of Christianity has been subdued in the last few hundred years, at times even suppressed. In Christian mysticism the word 'contemplation' is used rather than 'meditation'. Meditation methods of the Eastern kind we have described in this chapter may still be found in the Greek and Russian Orthodox Churches: for example, the repetition of the Jesus Prayer or Prayer of the Heart, 'Lord Jesus Christ, have mercy on me'. The Christian Fathers linked repetition of this prayer with the rhythms of breathing. And the anonymous monk who wrote *The Cloud of Unknowing* in the fourteenth century was not unfamiliar with one of the techniques described above.

Take a short word, preferably of one syllable . . . the shorter the word the better, being more like the meaning of the Spirit: a word like 'God' or 'love'. Choose one which you like, or perhaps some other so long as it is of one syllable. And fix this word fast to your heart, so that it is always there come what may. It will be your shield and spear in peace and war alike. With this word you will suppress all thought under the cloud of forgetting.

There are psychological as well as religious interpretations of mystical experience, and it may be sought for reasons that are not religious.

The physiological and psychological effects of meditation are now known as never before. That relaxation and equanimity of mind are effects of meditation practice have been known for thousands of years, but when Westerners took up meditation in great number in the 1960s these effects became of special importance in view of the stress-beset nature of life in most Western societies, especially of urban life.

Meditation promotes self-control of one's inner world, a neglected area in the Western world. Meditation is mental hygiene, reducing anxiety and tension in the mind, and giving relief from the pressure of clamouring thoughts.

Because meditation can be effective in eliciting the relaxation response, it is now used by psychotherapists to treat patients suffering from anxiety, tension, phobias, nervousness and psychosomatic ailments. It reduces the stress attached to injury or disease.

Patients with mental problems in Japan are being helped by zazen while in the USA transcendental meditation has been used to treat many of the ailments and behavioural problems that benefit from other forms of relaxation therapy. Meditation has been successful in breaking drug addiction where other methods have failed.

These results are not due to any occult or mystical forces, but mainly due to the relaxation response.

As meditation alters consciousness, it has special usefulness in changing attitudes. It also ripens the mind and prepares the brain and nervous system for peak experiences: moments of delight and heightened gratitude for living that have the power to alter consciousness and to transform values.

General health and wellbeing are improved by meditation. It promotes emotional control and tranquillity. Interpersonal relations are improved, because the person meditating is more relaxed, more tolerant, more accepting, and more open to change. And the feeling of mental calm that is induced by meditation tends to be carried into the hurly burly of everyday living. This may be advanced by the conscious practice of mindfulness of what is happening in the here and now, which will be discussed in the next chapter.

# 9 Meditation in Everyday Life

Meditation is not a practice which is restricted to twenty minutes or so sitting meditation daily. In all the major meditative traditions, sitting meditation alternates with meditative awareness in the ordinary activities of everyday living.

Coming out of sitting meditation and resuming normal activities marks the transition from awareness focused within to open and more general awareness, though the practice of 'just sitting' described in the preceding chapter is a sitting exercise in open awareness.

A Chinese Buddhist text says of this transition:

> Entry and exit should be both orderly for then
> The states of coarse and fine do not impair each other.
> This is like a horse that's tamed
> At your will to stay or go.

The practice of sitting meditation takes both the meditator and his nervous system from gross to subtle awareness and activity. Sitting meditation should be brought to an end in such a way that the transition to active life will be gradual and retain the feeling of relaxation and of poised awareness for as long as possible. Sit for a minute or two becoming aware of the external world before opening your eyes; then take another minute or two sitting motionless with your eyes open. These two to four minutes will be similar to the experience of 'just sitting' meditation. Then unfold your legs and stretch them slowly while continuing easy awareness. Be aware of a few easy in and out breaths, then rise to your feet slowly and go about your activities.

## MOBILE MEDITATION

Any natural carry over of meditative awareness from sitting meditation into active consciousness should be supported by periods of meditation during the active course of each day.

Just as head to toes relaxation lying down can be carried beneficially into everyday activities, so, too, you should carry the poised attention, awareness and attitude that is meditation into your everyday life: into the market place, the office, the factory, the commuter train, and so on. Also onto the playing field, the athletic track, the tennis court, the golf course, according to your leisure pursuits.

And just as attention wanders during sitting meditation and is brought back easily to the meditation object as many times as is necessary, so each time you become aware that you have ceased to be 'mindful' in mobile meditation you should return to poised attention, whatever you are doing.

This is the meditative practice which the Buddhists call mindfulness and bare attention, which the Zen Buddhists call mobile Zen, which the Taoists call flowing with the Tao, which the Sufis call self-remembering, which Krishnamurti calls choiceless awareness and which Christians call awareness of the presence of God. It is reverence for what you are doing for the Karma Yogin; Martin Heidegger's remembrance of existence; and Colin Wilson's sustained intentionality. Any differences there may be in these practices are of emotional tone rather than of essential attitude. Each is based on poised awareness of the here and now.

The practice of meditation in daily life is nowhere stronger than in Buddhism, being attributed to the Buddha himself. The terms 'mindfulness' and 'bare attention' are those I will be most using here.

# WHAT IS MINDFULNESS?

The Buddha taught that mindfulness is to 'see clearly on the spot that object which is *now*, while finding and living in a still, unmoving state of mind.' Bhikkhu Mangalo calls mindfulness 'recollection' and says it is 'quite simply, remembering to establish the attention with full awareness on the present, on the here and now.'

Nyanoponika Thera, a contemporary Buddhist monk, has written *The Heart of Buddhist Mindfulness: A Handbook of Mental Training Based on the Buddha's Way of Mindfulness*. He defines bare attention as 'the clear and single-minded awareness of what actually happens *to* us and *in* us, at the successive moments of awareness', and also as 'a bare and exact registering of the object'. We do not normally do this. Seeing things without labelling them or commenting on them inside the mind opens up a new world of perception. Nyanoponika Thera says that

the systematic cultivation of Right Mindfulness, as taught by the Buddha . . . still provides the most simple and direct, the most thorough and effective, method for training and developing the mind for its daily tasks and problems as well as for its highest aim: mind's own unshakable deliverance from greed, hatred, and delusion. . . . It is as applicable in the lands of the West as in the East; in the midst of life's turmoil as well as in the peace of the monk's cell.

Right Mindfulness is the seventh factor in the Buddhist Noble Eightfold Path. Right Meditation is the eighth factor.

The *Satipatthana Sutta*, an important text of the Pali canon, is also known as the 'Discourse on the Practice of Mindfulness'. The words are attributed to the Buddha. It opens and closes with the following words: 'There is one way, monks, for the purification of beings, for the overcoming of sorrows and grief, for the going down of sufferings and miseries, for winning the right path, for realising *nibbana*, that is to say, the four applications of mindfulness.' These applications are: (1) awareness of the body; (2) awareness of the feelings; (3) awareness of states of mind; (4) awareness of the contents of the mind. Awareness of the body begins with mindfulness of breathing – the sitting meditation described in the preceding chapter. Its benefits are described elsewhere in the Pali canon: 'This concentration of mind achieved through mindfulness of breathing, if cultivated and regularly practised, is peaceful and sublime, an unalloyed and happy state of mind that makes evil, unsalutary thoughts immediately cease and vanish wherever they arise.'

Formal sitting mindfulness is called main practice and the application of awareness to everyday living is called general practice.

As with sustaining awareness of a meditation object, an unbroken flow of meditative awareness in daily life is not as easy as it might at first appear. But now, as the focus of your awareness is simply everything that happens, thoughts and feelings will also be objects of bare attention. Bare attention of thoughts and feelings is not so immediately easy to sustain for short periods as mindfulness of sensory perceptions, but the ability comes with a little practice. It is this aspect of the Buddhist practice of mindfulness that is called *Vipassana* or insight meditation.

Detached awareness of the working of your mind gives insight into the mechanical nature of the ego, which Buddhists see as an illusory construct. When a Zen monk asked a master how to pacify his mind, the master replied: 'Show me your mind and I will pacify it.' The practice of insight meditation leads to understanding of the three characteristics of existence – impermanence, suffering and impersonality. Things of the inner and outer world are seen as impersonal processes – 'bare phenomena' (*suddha-dhamma*).

Bare attention weakens egocentricity, promotes detachment and reduces the stress in living. Nyanoponika Thera assures us that 'even its [bare attention's] casual application or routine use will show its liberating influence.'

Insight meditation is a practice of the Theravada or Southern School of Buddhism. There was a revival of the method at the beginning of this century due to the work of a Burmese monk, the Venerable U Narada Mahathera. In its direct confrontation with actuality, the overlapping of formal meditation and practice in everyday life, the transcending of conceptual thought, and in the emphasis on the present moment, this meditation based on mindfulness is close in spirit to Zen.


## MOBILE ZAZEN

At Zen monasteries and temples physical work (*samu*) is an important part of the training of the monk in the Zen way of life. Monks tend the gardens, sweep, clean and cook. They work with what looks like ritualistic poise: their inner attitude is poised also. Zen poise is not restricted to the zazen hall: meditation and everyday duties and relaxations are unified. The monks show respect for the tools and utensils they handle. Wastefulness and carelessness are viewed as an offence against life values. Food is stored, cooked and eaten with gratitude.

*Samu* is mobile zazen. It is Zen in action. Mindfulness is also brought to washing, dressing, eating, emptying bladder and bowels, and even, as mentioned earlier, to sleeping.

Christian monks give their labours a similar dignity, dedicating each task, however humble, to the glory of God. And as taught in the *Bhagavad Gita*, the Karma Yogin works mindfully without thought of the fruits of his actions.

Working – or playing – with a poised attitude gives a ritualistic look to physical activity. Things get done – and usually done well – but the doer looks and feels as if he has all the time in the world.


## THE TEA CEREMONY

The poised Zen attitude has had great influence on Japanese culture. An example is the relaxing tea ceremony, which the Japanese call *ch-no-yu*.

Father Joao Rodrigues (1562–1633), a Portuguese Jesuit who spent thirty years in Japan, reported back on the Japanese art of drinking tea. He observed that each utensil is 'as rustic, rough, completely unrefined and simple as nature made it, after the style of a solitary and rustic hermitage'. The purpose of the ceremony he said 'is to produce courtesy, politeness, modesty, exterior moderation, calmness, peace of body and soul without any pride or arrogance, fleeing from all ostentation, pomp, external grandeur, and magnificence.' This is very good as far as it goes. To the Zen-man the tea ceremony is also a ritual exercise in mindfulness: for all the surface calm it is concerned with the fundamental roots of existence.

If one sees the tea ceremony as an exercise in mindfulness, one sees its significance at the Zen level. There is an aesthetic factor.

Traditionally, antique utensils are used, but if you make tea and drink tea in the right spirit then mass-produced utensils would do. You may do it alone, or with family and friends.

In a way, the ceremony of drinking tea is already familiar to most British people, wherever they are in the world. They may not think of it in the terms used by the Japanese, but they are familiar with the tea-drinking of comfort, of solace, of reconciliation, of recovery after shock or disaster, of recuperation after hard physical work, and so on. Each social class in Britain has its characteristic tea-drinking ritual.

The samurai used the tea-drinking ceremony to calm the body and to empty the mind of thought before battle. The skill of the great Japanese swordsman is associated with the 'no mind' (*mushin* or *munen*) state of Zen.

The mindfulness exercise includes the preparation of the tea as much as its drinking. Making tea, drinking it, and conversing lightly with friends takes place within a psychic atmosphere for which Suzuki coined the word 'psychosphere'. The surroundings are simple, even austere. The room is small, in semidarkness. The participants talk in soft voices or sit silently listening to the sound of boiling water in the kettle on the charcoal fire or watching the wisps of smoke from the spout. Sipping the tea, every movement is mindful. The atmosphere and the mindfulness combine to produce a state of tranquil passivity. Making tea and drinking tea become meditation.

## SPONTANEITY AND FREEDOM

It should be remembered that Zen was the religion of the samurai, and may be thought of in connection with *kendo* (the Way of the Sword) and self-defence systems like judo and aikido as well as with the tea ceremony and flower arrangement. One of the fascinations of Zen is its combination of strength and delicacy.

Zen meditation builds up the concentrative power called *joriki*. Joriki is spiritual power, giving self-mastery and freedom from the push and pull of the emotions. It assists the maturing that leads to the enlightenment-awakening of satori (also called *kensho*). It is applied in moment-to-moment experiences of bare attention and is associated with the state of thought-cleared but powerful mind needed by the Zen swordsman.

Bare attention is awareness without judgement or any comment. It has directness, objectivity and strength. Krishnamurti is against systematized meditation but he recommends 'experiencing what is without naming', which he calls 'choiceless awareness'. This includes watching your thoughts. If the mind is looked at with 'choiceless awareness', Krishnamurti says, then of its own accord, having seen the totality of its own conditioning, it will become perfectly still.

Mindfulness is sometimes described as attention that is like two arrows side by side – one pointing outwards at an object and the other pointing back to the subject. Part of the mindful person stays aware of himself or herself.

Mindfulness may also be described as a state in which one is wholly present and wholly attending in any situation and so able to respond alertly and appropriately in it. In Zen, mindfulness – mobile zazen – leads to something similar or identical with Krishnamurti's stilled mind. This is *mushin* or *munen*, which may be translated as 'no-mind-ness'. This state may be understood most clearly as seen in the perfected Zen swordsman. Worth reading on this subject are the two chapters on 'Zen and Swordsmanship' in D. T. Suzuki's *Zen and Japanese Culture*.

In advanced Zen action – that stemming from the no-mind

state – appropriate action comes spontaneously, as the result of long physical, mental and spiritual training. This should not be confused with 'mechanicalness', which is accompanied by a dull state of consciousness, as can be witnessed in a mechanical performance of work or sport. If a sportsman's movements are described as 'mechanical', it means that his movements are laboured and lack life. In contrast, the reflexes of the Zen swordsman in the state of no-mind are wonderfully quick and vitally alive; the state has an alert brightness and a sense of freedom not known in ordinary consciousness.

The training of the Zen swordsman is in the Zen Way as well as in the psychophysical skills of swordsmanship. The goal is to drop ego-consciousness and to act spontaneously from the state of *mushin*. The perfected Zen swordsman stands in poised posture, is differentially relaxed yet full of energy, balanced and alert. In early training he is taught to centre in the tanden about two inches below the navel, but in advanced training the mind 'abides nowhere' and consciousness fills the whole body, so that his arms and his feet can move instantaneously. The swordsman is 'open on all sides', and it is important that the flow of the mind (and attention) should not stop. For the mind to 'stop' even momentarily on the opponent's sword or on any other place could be a moment of weakness that brings defeat. A definition of Zen enlightenment is 'awakening the mind without its abiding anywhere'. That is why a sport can also be a 'Way', a path to mystical awakening.

D. T. Suzuki says that the training of the Zen swordsman is a practical application of the old Taoist doctrine of 'doing by not doing' (*wu-wei*). Lao Tzu's *Tao Te Ching*, the most beautiful text of philosophical Taoism, may be looked upon as the greatest manual of poised living.

Suzuki says: 'Zen is concerned with a movement of instantaneity in which the flint emits a spark when it strikes steel.' Zen masters, when they perceive that psychological maturity has ripened, will trigger the enlightenment experience (satori) in a pupil by sharply calling his name or even striking him with a stick. Enlightenment often comes through hearing a sharp sound or seeing something bright or colourful. Zazen and other Zen training ripens the mind for the experience, which transforms consciousness.

Note that even though the Zen swordsman's mind keeps moving in harmony with its nature, there is nevertheless a still centre to experience. An analogy is drawn in Zen with the reflection of the moon which is set in motion by flowing water though the moon itself is there in the sky, whole, clear and serene.

It hardly needs saying that this Oriental attitude does not mean that there is no need for thought. Life is lived more in bare attention to the present, but thought, including thought of past and future, occurs when appropriate. When unnecessary 'head-talk' is reduced, it is found that essential thinking becomes more powerful and productive.

Work or any other activity performed as meditation or as an act of reverence or gratitude for living is valued for itself and so receives devoted attention. Though results are not thought about, the outcome is usually effective productivity or satisfying artistic creation. This is because there is no straining for results, no burdensome thoughts of 'I must succeed'. The Zen archer may be congratulated whether he hits the target or not, when he has demonstrated the artless art of 'shooting that is non-shooting'. 'Wonderful what a two goal lead can do,' says the football commentator. 'Now that the pressure is off, they (the winning side) are demonstrating all their fluent skills.' Winning or losing, the 'perfect man' of Taoism and Zen performs with poise and natural ease and grace because for him the pressure is always off. He is free of unnecessary muscular contractions and of egocentric burdens.

If we are interested in exploring the most advanced developments of psychophysical poise, the concept and practice of Taoist/Zen spontaneity will attract us. I hope that it is clear from the above few paragraphs that no-mind-ness bears no resemblance to 'mindless violence' or 'mindless stupidity' and similar terms. It is the flower of spiritual training that requires great subtlety and dedication.

The spontaneity of Zen has been abused by people who have ignored the discipline and the poise of mind and character required, and misconstrued the term as meaning licentiousness. Many of the 'beat generation' in the USA were guilty of this lax understanding of Zen, though the movement produced a few figures, like the poet Gary Snyder, with real understanding of Zen in letter and spirit. On this matter, see Alan Watts's 'Beat Zen, Square Zen, and Zen', published in *This Is It and Other Essays on Zen and Spiritual Experience*.

When the Zen approach to living is adequately understood, words like no-mind, fluidity, no-abiding mind, non-stopping mind, instantaneity, spontaneity, freedom and purposelessness will not be seen negatively but as pointers to relaxed and poised living of a high order. Taoist and Zen art expresses the beauty of freedom of the spirit. In Eastern eyes, too much purpose in a work of art destroys its spontaneity, beauty and significance. Art, too, is a way to poised living and enlightenment.

## FINDING LIFE MEANINGFUL

When you wash, dress, eat, drink, work, play and create in a state of psychophysical poise and mindfulness, then every moment of living becomes meaningful. This is something for each reader to experience for himself or herself.

Psychiatrists, psychoanalysts and psychotherapists today face a new development. The majority of their patients do not suffer from the sexual guilt and repression seen and written about by Freud and his colleagues. The main anxiety problem today is finding life lacking in meaning. New schools of psychotherapy – existentialist, humanistic, and so on – represent a third force in psychology (the other two are Freudianism and behaviourism) to meet the psychological and spiritual malaise of our times. The causes have often been discussed: alienation in a technological civilization, comfort and affluence, decline in spiritual belief, and so on.

A major problem today is that most people, to put it bluntly, think too much. Using the language of general semantics, they ail to separate two levels of abstraction – the verbal and the non-verbal. Most daily 'self-talk' and 'head-chatter' is negative, unnecessary, unproductive, and destructive of human happiness and fulfilment. In addition, people muffle and distort their sensory perceptions by bringing verbal commentary into what should be non-verbal experiences.

'Rose is a rose is a rose is a rose,' wrote Gertrude Stein. Language is man's greatest evolutionary achievement, and there is nothing wrong with thinking about roses or writing poems about roses. But there *is* something wrong if few people look at a rose, smell a rose, or touch a rose just as it is – with bare attention, without verbalizing.

The beauty of a rose might hold your attention without thinking about it for some seconds at least, but try doing it with a teacup, a pencil, a blade of grass, or a thumbnail. It is very difficult to sustain bare awareness for more than a few seconds, but with practice you should be able to do it for some minutes. The experience of seeing objects cleanly at a non-verbal level without word and thought associations is amazingly refreshing and meaningful. It is a way of instantly injecting new energy, clarity and meaning into consciousness. Yet the object selected for the exercise may seem trivial at the verbal level of abstraction.

Colin Wilson says in some of his books that he can make life feel more meaningful by repeatedly staring at a pencil. There is no need to strain the eyes by staring – like the Zen swordsman's mind, the eyes are designed to keep their areas of greatest sensitivity in continual movement. Stop. Look. Look with bare attention, staying on the non-verbal level. Just look.

Repeat the exercise with your other senses, using other objects. Just touch, closing your eyes. Close your eyes again and just hear. One way to enjoy music is to listen to it while influencing your feelings with thoughts about the composer, the emotions aroused by the music, and so on. But another way is to just listen to the sound, with your eyes closed, without verbalizing. For many music lovers this gives a whole new experience.

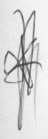

It will be seen now why the practice of mindfulness is a mental hygiene, and a method of psychotherapy. If you are imprisoned by your verbal thinking, bare attention brings delight and freedom. If you stop wrapping up your perceptions in bundles of old rags – accumulated thought-words – you will discover meaning in daily concrete experiences, in the little everyday activities of life as well as in the important and dramatic. There will be meaning and refreshment in gazing at a patch of sunlight on a bedroom wall, the corner of a roof, the fall of rain, a fried egg, and a soup tin (without any help from the art of Andy Warhol).

Art does help us to look at familiar things in unfamiliar ways, just as novelists and poets help us see everyday things and human relationships in a fresh light. 'Old Earth Man' John Cowper Powys wrote lengthily, often repetitively, but always zestfully on this theme. In particular he recommended contemplation of the natural elements earth, water, air and fire. Even if you live in a city bedsitter, you can have earth in a windowbox or flowerpot, water in a vase, air from a window, and fire from a match or gas stove. A form of mindfulness is a tenet of Powys's practical philosophy. Though he was in his own way a master of English prose, it is of the old wordy style with long, complex sentences: modern taste prefers a sharper thrust.

Colin Wilson wrote that when he reads John Cowper Powys's books he can 'hear Aunt Agatha's knitting-kneedles clicking'; but he clearly finds much to admire in his ideas about sounding the depths of meaning in the world about us. In a magazine article about Colin Wilson, he was quoted as saying that a ray of sunlight striking breakfast cornflakes may provide a peak experience of the Proustian kind that convinces us that life is not just a series of dreary obstacles. He had seen life that way in his teens and twice contemplated suicide, but peak experiences had totally changed his outlook on life.

Peak experiences are more likely to occur in the person who learns how to sustain bare attention at will. And bare attention is easier to practise for the person who has learned to let go from muscular and mental tension and to quieten the mind. Tension 'static' in the mind and thought-chatter prevents mindfulness; relaxation encourages it. Mindfulness has an element of detachment, which saves wear and tear on the nervous system and raises the stress threshold.

The power of mindfulness increases the more you separate the non-verbal level from the verbal. It then breaks up our tired habituated perception and replaces our dull automatized experience with a new fresh enjoyment of the familiar. Details of the world about us will be noticed again with a freshness perhaps not known or rarely known since childhood. This occurs if attention is given to the first striking of the flint in perception, which Zen Buddhists call the first *nen*. The second nen is the reflecting action of consciousness. When there is perception without reaction, experience is bright and fresh. Brightness blazes in the peak Zen experience of satori or *kensho*, for which Zen meditation prepares and ripens the mind. Subject–object duality is transcended, as is the sense of separation between mind and external universe. This is the 'awakening' in which 'one sees into one's true nature'.

Some books on meditation have listed satori as the Zen equivalent of the Yoga samadhi, but there is an inaccuracy here. Satori occurs on coming out of the pure contentless consciousness of samadhi. The external environment breaks in vividly on pure awareness, triggered maybe by a single sharp sensory impression. Zen literature contains many stories about enlightenment occurring in this way. When the mind has been ripened by meditation, the apple falls. One monk experienced *kensho* when sweeping the ground with a broom – the broom flicked a stone against a bomboo plant, the sound triggering the 'explosion' or 'turn over' of consciousness that is such a valuable experience that life is usually transformed by it. The experience fades but is usually repeated on other occasions, and its quality suffuses ordinary consciousness. The main aim of Zen is to live in permanent higher consciousness, which is also the supreme attainment for aspirants in other mystical traditions.

Katsuki Sekida distinguishes between absolute and positive samadhi. Absolute samadhi is pure consciousness of the kind experienced in formal sitting meditation – 'you don't know you're there, but you know you've been'. Positive samadhi is the first nen perception in satori, in lesser intensity, but still full of brightness and meaning, in mindfulness free of verbalization.

Positive samadhi may occur following a period of concentrated brain work: the intellect switches off and sense perceptions are heightened. The experience is not fully satisfactory because of the mental fatigue. It may also occur through reaction to chemicals: drinking alcohol, smoking 'pot', and so on. Again de-automatization could account for the newness of the vision, but the person who takes alcohol or drugs risks dangers to body and mind from habitual use of chemicals that alter consciousness. A third way that perceptions may be heightened with the clarity associated with positive samadhi is on a clear morning following deeply refreshing sleep. T. E. Lawrence described such an experience in the desert – a 'clear dawn that woke up the senses with the sun', while his intellect stayed asleep.

Meditation, whether formal or mobile, is practical training in freshening awareness. Heightened perception often follows concentrative sitting meditation and often occurs during the 'open' meditation we have discussed in this chapter.

## HABITUATION AND DIS-HABITUATION

Japanese neuropsychiatrists Tomio Hirai and A. Kasamatsu made an electroencephalographic study of Zen meditation. One experiment was to test the orienting response to a repeated click by two groups – one of 'ordinary' people and one of Zen priests. A click was repeated each fifteen seconds in a soundproof room. A normal response would be for a subject to become used to the click and for the electrical response in the brain to decrease progressively with the first few clicks and then be tuned right out of awareness. This happened with all of the control group. But not with the Zen priests. The clicks went on for five minutes. The Zen men responded to all the clicks in the same way: there was no habituation. Their brains responded to the last click just as they had done to the first click.

Another way of putting this is that the Zen men did not allow repetition to stale their response, which stayed fresh. Similar results were found in Indian Yogins who during meditation were able to cut out all external stimuli from awareness. Dr Robert E. Ornstein, in his contribution to *On the Psychology of Meditation*, says that concentrative 'shutting down' meditation of the Yogic kind leads to 'opening up' of awareness afterwards and he would expect no habituation. He would also expect dis-habituation during 'opening up' meditation like the Zen 'just sitting' and mindfulness in everyday life.

The points we have been discussing open up possibilities for experiencing our external world anew every day. And to see things freshly is to enjoy them with an innocent eye. Taking a dog for a walk could be as enjoyable for us, every time, as it is for the dog. And those readers who like playing gramophone records will know the disappointment that comes when one enjoys the first few playings of a record, only for the fresh impact to progressively fade with each further playing. The best music has the power to burgeon in our minds again and again. However, tastes for composers change and the works of certain composers may easily lose appeal. Understanding of the working of habituation and of dis-habituation can provide a means of freshly hearing and enjoying music. One way to begin has already been mentioned: listen to the pattern of sounds – on the non-verbal level of abstraction.

It strikes me that listening to a personal collection of gramophone records could become a Way, a form of development in the art of living. One factor would be an existentialist approach to music of the kind which Colin Wilson began in *The Brandy of the Damned*. Listening to records would also become a method of meditation – which it already is for most music lovers. The best way to listen is in poised meditative posture with eyes closed and staying perfectly still.

Before leaving this question of how to give awareness a fresher quality, you may like to try performing everyday tasks like shaving, putting on trousers or tights, and so on in a different order to that which has become habitual. Start shaving on the other side of your face, or pulling on the other leg of trousers or tights first. 'The Robot' suffers at least a momentary defeat. He is useful so long as he works when we want him to on the jobs that we want him to do. If he dominates our lives so much that consciousness becomes dull and lifeless, it is time to start taking measures to come to life again, including mindfulness in everyday living.

## NON-ATTACHMENT

Mindfulness is relaxing because it helps us slow down or, more accurately perhaps, have the subjective experience of slowing down. We will resemble the skilled footballer in this, who never seems hurried, who 'makes time' for himself and who 'creates space' for himself, but in whom 'slowness' is an illusion.

Mindfulness is relaxing also because it 'creates space' between oneself and what is experienced, including one's own thoughts and feelings. This is the element of non-attachment in poised meditation. This is a psychological state and not asceticism. But you can relax and open up awareness to more things when the clamour of desires is eliminated or at least toned down. When the ego is rampant, there is no time to allow the singing of a bird or the appreciation of a poem into the consciousness. In mindfulness consciousness becomes like a mirror that accepts everything but clings to nothing.

This aspect of mindfulness is stressed by Nyanoponika Thera in *The Heart of Buddhist Mindfulness*, p. 43, when he explains the value of bare attention for liberating the mind:

The suggestion is proffered to the reader that he may try, at first for a few test days, to keep as well as he can to an attitude of Bare Attention towards people, inanimate environment and the various happenings of the day. By doing so he will soon feel how much more harmoniously such days are passing compared with those when he gave in to the slightest stimulus for interfering by deed, word, emotion or thought. As if protected by an invisible armour against the banalities and importunities of the outer world, one will walk through such days serenely and content, with an exhilarating feeling of ease and freedom. It is as if, from the unpleasant closeness of a hustling and noisy crowd, one has escaped to the silence and seclusion of a hill top, and, with a sigh of relief, is looking down on the noise and bustle below. It is the peace and happiness of detachment which will thus be experienced. By thus stepping back from things and men, one's attitude towards them will even become friendlier, because those tensions will be lacking which so often arise from interfering, desire, aversion, or other forms of self-reference. Life will become a good deal easier, and one's inner and outer world more spacious. In addition, we will notice that the world goes on quite well without our earlier amount of intervention, and that we ourselves are all the better for such a restraint. How many entanglements will not be avoided, and how many problems will not solve themselves without our contribution! Hereby Bare Attention shows visibly the benefit of abstaining from karmic action, be it good or evil, i.e. from a world-building, sorrow-creating activity. Bare Attention schools us in the art of letting go, weans us from busy-ness and from habitual interfering.

The inner distance from things, men and from ourselves, as obtained temporarily and partially by Bare Attention, shows us, by our own experience, the possibility of finally winning **perfect** detachment and the happiness resulting from it. . . .

# 10 Relaxation and the Mind's Reaches

## USING AUTO-SUGGESTION

About sixty years ago Emile Coué wrote: 'To make good suggestions, it is absolutely necessary to do it *without effort* . . . the use of the *will* . . . must be entirely put aside.'

By 'good suggestions' Coué was referring to effective auto-suggestion. A suggestion has to be passively accepted for there to be a chance of it working.

For some years in the 1920s auto-suggestion became something of a craze in Europe and America. Coué used auto-suggestion therapeutically at a clinic in Nancy, France, and for a time received considerable publicity: his general auto-suggestion 'Every day, in every way, I am getting better and better' remains well known to this day. Then his ideas suddenly died out. Probably insufficient people understood what was required – passive acceptance of the suggestions.

The fact remains that certain states of mind are propitious to implanting suggestions in the subconscious or unconscious mind that will take root and tend to be realized without the person doing anything about it. The mind's own powers take over and set about realizing the ideas, as long as they are realistic and the suggestions have been given in an appropriate form.

The states of mind most suitable for passive acceptance of verbal or visual suggestions are:

1  The state of hypnotic trance
2  The hypnogogic state that precedes sleep

3  The state of light sleep. Some writers say that about one
   hour after going to sleep is a good time for sleep suggestion
4  The state of deep relaxation and mental calm

Of these four states of mind, the fourth is the most easily
utilized by every person. Some people cannot reach the state of
hypnosis, or only with the aid of a hypnotist. The hypnogogic
state is characterized by floating images and one can easily
become lost in them, passing into sleep before adequately
implanting the chosen suggestion formula. During sleep the
suggestions have to be given by another person or your own
recorded voice. There are no problems with the calm and
relaxed state in which there is clear awareness. It should be said,
however, that states 1 to 3 may work well for some people, and
that unless there is conscious or unconscious unease about self-
hypnosis, the procedure of induction will probably induce state
4, if not the state of hypnotic trance.
It is difficult to differentiate between some of the states of
deep relaxation. Auto-suggestion may sometimes be auto-
hypnosis, and what is believed to be auto-hypnosis may sometimes be auto-suggestion. Autogenic training is often described
as a form of training in self-hypnosis, but this writer and many
other people are not convinced that it is on all occasions for all
people. For many people, I believe, the autogene state is deep
relaxation and mental calm induced by verbal suggestion –
induced, that is, by self-suggestion. There are experts on
hypnosis who say there is no such separate state: it is all a matter
of auto-suggestion. Bring in the state of meditation and the
alternatives become prolonged and tedious. Some people
experienced in the practice both of self-hypnosis and of meditation say they cannot differentiate between the alleged two
states. On the other hand . . . but why go on? Perhaps brainwave biofeedback will come up with some answers. Biofeedback researchers have begun this work, but the position is still
mostly confusing. Meanwhile, let each of us find the deep
relaxation method or methods that suit us and, if so minded,
utilize the state of mind for passive reception of verbal

suggestions and/or visual images aimed at improving health, changing habits, attaining greater confidence or making better use of our skills and potentialities.

When the mind is calm, suggestions that are realistic and simply and directly worded tend to be taken in by the unconscious, which sets about realizing them.

Direct, positive suggestions work best. Better to say 'I will feel energetic' than 'I will not feel tired'. In phrasing suggestions, avoid negative words like 'not', 'can't', 'don't', and 'won't'. But don't bully the unconscious – though it sometimes works for very submissive types. Say 'I can' rather than 'I will' or 'I must'. Another way of avoiding forcing commands on the unconscious is to give it time to effect change by using words like 'soon' or 'begin to',

Repeat the phrases inwardly, slowly and steadily, four or five times. *Think* the words; don't subvocalize – that is, don't move your vocal muscles. Thinking is intimate and is in the mind.

It has been discovered that visualized images powerfully reinforce verbal suggestions. So see yourself behaving as you suggest you will become and behave. Coué, who deserves higher regard than he usually receives, observed: 'When the imagination and the will are in conflict, the imagination always wins.' The important thing, therefore, is to harness the power of the imagination and make it work for us.

During auto-suggestion the conscious will should be in abeyance. Coué discovered that ideas are seeds and tend towards realization when passively received. Willing a wart to go away will have no effect, but when a child with a wart is given some money and told that the wart has been bought, this old folk remedy often works, because the child's unconscious has accepted the suggestion.

Another insight that Coué had was 'the law of reversed effort'. We are all familiar with it. A good example is how if we try to get to sleep we cannot – but when we give up trying and relax sleep comes. The same is true about trying to relax. Relaxation comes through not trying, by letting it happen. Biofeedback researchers who asked people to see if they could make a finger become warmer were surprised to find finger temperatures dropping. This happened because the subjects were trying too hard to raise finger temperature. When they substituted passive awareness, they succeeded. Coué would have understood immediately the cause of the earlier failure.

## TRUE WILL

There is growing interest in awakening latent powers, such as those investigated in parapsychology, and the role of relaxation in the awakening and testing of these powers is insufficiently understood or appreciated. Relaxation is an essential preliminary to the manifestation of most so-called paranormal powers. It has a key part to play by pacifying the conscious mind and will, so that the deep-seated true will may emerge. This true will, effortless because powered by the mighty engines of the unconscious, crops up frequently through the centuries in treatises on magic, occultism and myticism. It is familiar to the poet and to the artist, as well as to the mystic.

Furthermore, relaxation is the essence of the 'peak experience' – those moments of transcendental freedom and ecstasy which Professor Abraham H. Maslow found to be frequent in one type of psychologically healthy, self-actualizing person. Maslow, a pioneer of humanistic psychology, showed that 'peaks' were characteristic of mentally healthy men and women and need not be divorced from normal consciousness. 'What is the Tao?' a great Zen master was asked. 'Ordinary mind is the Tao,' was the reply. Whether or not you wish to use the word 'mystical' to describe peak experiences depends on how one defines this elusive term.

In descriptions of mystical experience from the voices or pens of the great mystics one discerns a letting go from the ego with all its tension knots, its desires and anxieties, an opening up, a stepping out into blissful freedom. In short, classic mystical experience may be viewed as the ultimate relaxation experience.

## COLIN WILSON

If you read the full output of this zestful writer, you will find growing awareness of the role of 'true will' and 'true relaxation' in increasing the range and intensity of consciousness, his central concern. This understanding was fully apparent to me on reading his books of the seventies. Though the word 'relaxation' does not appear in the indexes of *The Occult* (1971), *New Pathways in Psychology* (1972) and *Mysteries* (1978), I rectified the omissions in my own copies. When I added the word 'relaxation' to the index of *Mysteries*, I wrote down nineteen page references: I also added entries for 'mental poise' and 'true will'.

In *Mysteries,* Colin Wilson wrote: 'It is relatively easy to "glide" into freedom – or some small degree of freedom – in moments of relaxation' (p. 441). These moments are accompanied by 'the feeling of *expanded powers*'.

Colin Wilson is saying that by letting go and opening up we increase the amount of freedom we have from the stranglehold of habit, which he calls 'the robot'; we become more conscious, more vitally alive, and gain access to a wider sense of reality. We experience the heightened sense of meaningfulness in living as the 'real me'. Colin Wilson uses the terms 'real me', 'real I', and 'real you' the way Zen Buddhists speak of 'true nature' and 'Buddha nature'.

'True relaxation . . . is an influx of meaning, as if the brain was a battery "on charge",' he wrote in *New Pathways in Psychology* (p. 120) and he correctly points out (p. 258) that 'genuine relaxation' is the essence of the peak experience. In the practice of mindfulness or bare attention, which I described in chapter 9, the sense of meaning is 'switched on', leading to insight and more peak experiences.

## ALTERED STATES OF CONSCIOUSNESS

Some people feel uneasy about altered states of consciousness, as though they are something strange that could not possibly apply to them. But we all have fluctuations in the quality of consciousness. There is a change when we daydream or dream in sleep; taking an alcoholic drink alters consciousness; so does missing a meal or eating a heavy dinner. Listening to music or reading poetry produces a qualitative change; so does letting deep relaxation happen or meditating using a traditional technique. Consciousness alters in peak experiences – those precious moments in life when we feel carried out of ourselves by some transport of delight or ecstasy. It is a matter of awareness: states of consciousness are states of awareness. These states may or may not represent something of significance beyond themselves; but the changes are real and may be experienced for oneself.

Masters of the esoteric psychologies say that what passes for consciousness in our ordinary waking state is a poor and dim experience, a kind of waking sleep in contrast with what is possible in higher states of consciousness. These masters may vary in their interpretations of the experience, but there is agreement about the basic experience *per se*.

The psychological fact that these states of consciousness exist should be taken into account – especially as they appear to represent greater freedom from one's conditioning, greater relaxation and greater poise.

During sitting meditation one is aware of various things – sounds, body position, skin sensations, internal sensations, the slight movement of the breathing muscles, feelings, and the appearance in the mind of thoughts and images. There is also, repeatedly, as foreground figure, the mantra or whatever psychological device is being used to help quieten the mind.

## PURE BEING

Something else happens in consciousness. Its quality changes: becomes finer, subtler, purer. There are periods of pure being, existence, or consciousness when the mind is like an illuminated cinema screen when no film is passing between the lens and the light source. In these periods there is no sense of time passing and no experience really to remember. During them breathing stops or nearly stops. Body sensation drops off, giving the 'off sensation'. These periods of pure being may last seconds or minutes, the meditator cannot be sure; but as he or she leaves the clear state of mind and a thought, image, feeling or sense impression is coming in, there is a subtle awareness of leaving the clear state.

The Sanskrit word used in the East for this pure state of consciousness is samadhi. Maharishi Mahesh Yogi calls it 'pure being', the Zen writer Katsuki Sekida calls it samadhi and also 'pure existence'. Biofeedback researchers into meditation link the clear state with the production of alpha waves in the brain.

## WHAT'S THE POINT?

Many people ask: what's the point of making your mind a blank?

Well, switching off the contents of consciousness for even a few seconds, even the brief gap between two thoughts, is mental relaxation. With experience in meditation the periods of clear consciousness become longer – one is surprised that the minutes of meditation have passed so quickly – and the after-effect is a great sense of mental relaxation and a bright clarity of mind. The body, too, has relaxed deeply and many of its physiological functions have slowed down.

## LUCID LIVING

There is a further stage to report. The pure relaxing quality of samadhi, the quality of the ground of consciousness, is carried into normal waking consciousness and fuses with it. There is a period of about ten minutes, which shows on the EEG as alpha waves, when meditation consciousness lingers. Then' the afterglow fades away, but perhaps not entirely. Meditators who have meditated perhaps twice daily for a considerable number of months or years may report that they are able to retain the feeling of relaxing meditation consciousness throughout the minute-to-minute activity of ordinary waking consciousness for long periods, perhaps even permanently.

Maharishi Mahesh Yogi likens the process to dipping cloth into dye. The cloth is spread out in the sun and dries, then dipped and again dried in the sun. The cloth becomes more and more deeply coloured by the dips into the dye and finally is fully saturated by it.

Dips into pure being during transcendental meditation, Maharishi Mahesh Yogi says, end up with your everyday consciousness having a permanent quality of purity and poise.

You can help the suffusion of normal waking consciousness with the peaceful and stress-resistant quality through the practice of mindfulness in everyday living, and through the other methods described in this book for the cultivation of poised living. Monitoring your brainwaves during and after meditation may be a useful way of learning to retain the feeling of meditative mental relaxation for longer periods than the usual ten minutes or so of afterglow.

## A FIFTH STATE OF CONSCIOUSNESS?

If you believe these alterations in consciousness represent a hierarchy of states of consciousness, then the pure consciousness of meditation may be looked upon as a fourth state of consciousness, a pure substrate without content. Preceding this state in the scale are dreamless sleep, dreaming sleep, and ordinary waking consciousness. When ordinary waking consciousness (third state) is fused with clear meditation consciousness (fourth state), the result is fifth state of consciousness. The cloth is fully dyed and may be worn in everything you do without fear of its fading. The position is more complicated, for the suffusion will be mild at first and perhaps not sustained in everything that is done for some time. Peak mystical experiences are most likely to produce a powerful transformation of ordinary waking consciousness, as in the Zen satori, for which the mind is ripened by frequent periods of samadhi. Even then the experience needs to be repeated and deepened.

For some readers the whole idea of states of higher and lower consciousness may seem fanciful and pretentious, even in the straightforward way I have described it, free from religious associations and terminology. But it should be acceptable to such readers to see the process as the relaxation response, with its slowing down of physiological processes, quietening the nervous system so that day-to-day living becomes more relaxed. Transcendental meditation's researchers say that meditation does produce changes in the nervous sytem. It may also be seen that as skill in psychophysical relaxation develops through use of any of the methods described in this book, you become more relaxed in all of living. Methods of carrying relaxation into active living have been described, additional to the carryover effect from deep relaxation practice.

Through the relaxation techniques described in this book, you are likely to become more relaxed in all that you do, including sleeping. Attitudes, too, are changed. You are likely to find that your life has acquired a whole new quality – depth, breadth, even beauty. Being becomes more important than having, and being values more important than deficiency values (discussed in the following chapter).

Dr Herbert Benson equates the relaxation response with the experience of meditation consciousness, but describes a physiological response. Beyond that lies the age-old belief in stages of mystical consciousness. Many people find their altered states of consciousness so significant that they see them either as part of a hierarchy of states of consciousness relating to man's evolutionary development or as stages on a mystical and religious Way that leads to union with Cosmic Mind, God, or an impersonal or quasi-personal Absolute.

It is possible also to take an approach which says: consciousness clearly can be altered in certain ways by healthy drugless methods, and the effect is relaxing, enriching and fulfilling and so worthy of my cultivation and exploration while I remain open and uncommitted about religious and other interpretations.

# 11 The Art of Poised Living

In the preceding chapters practical techniques were described for more relaxed and happier living. This concluding chapter outlines the strategy for their use and gives a picture of the likely attitudes, psychology, philosophy, and world view of the man or woman realizing a poised life.

## STRATEGY FOR LIVING

The art of poised living is grounded in the practice of techniques of general relaxation and of sitting meditation, and the application of muscular relaxation (differential relaxation) and mindfulness (mobile meditation) in active everyday living. Ordinary waking consciousness will become more relaxed and poised due to the daily use of the above techniques, both involuntary and voluntary influences being at work. Poised attitudes will be produced as the outcome of the influence of techniques of relaxation and poise on the emotions, thought and nervous system. They may also be cultivated as the result of a conscious decision based on their self-validating worth.

An example of the involuntary influence is the way poised outer posture tends to shape a harmonious inner posture. Attitudes are an inner stance directed towards the world, other people and oneself. Posture is not just the disposal of limbs and trunk in a particularly wellbalanced way, but, as the *Concise Oxford Dictionary* tell us, 'carriage, attitude of body *or* mind;

condition, state'. A whole way of life is implied in the words 'poised posture' – poised attitudes as well as poised standing, sitting, and acting. Poise is the stance we take towards the world and other people.

When the body is poised, then it can be easily and naturally used in work and in play, in lifting and in carrying, in walking and in running, in driving a car and in giving birth. The voluntary aspect is the cognitive factor of choosing the right actions for conserving energy and using the minimum effort for the maximum effect.

Relaxed muscles and relaxed attitudes combine to increase the ease and the pleasure of home life, work and play. More energy is available for use and is used more economically yet more tellingly. Health improves and you will not be the personality type prone to major diseases – the heart-attack type, the nervous breakdown type, the cancer type and the stress-disease type. Poised living is a strategy for survival.

Relaxed attitudes take the sting out of the great modern stressors – competition, complexity and change. Achievement is enjoyed for its own sake and the rat race is left to the rats; complexity is found interesting rather than overwhelming and change is accepted as the law of life without which there would be stagnation and neither variety nor growth, no day and night, no seasons . . . in short, an inconceivable, monotonous and soul-destroying world.

As relaxed living becomes a reality there will be no need for chemical aids to relaxation, such as tranquillizers, drugs, tobacco and alcohol – though beer and wine may be enjoyed for their own sakes. You will find that many things are being done and enjoyed for their own sakes.

## POISED ATTITUDES AND FREEDOM

Attitudes are important because they determine emotions and behaviour. The influence of psychophysical relaxation, poised posture, breathing and meditation will shape poised attitudes and encourage recognition of their self-validating worth.

Attitudes may be chosen, and once chosen acted upon: they shape life styles. The choice may be made on rational and indeed commonsense grounds. The wisdom of certain attitudes may be arrived at through quiet contemplation of what is involved, taking a broad perspective.

The aim of poised living is greater freedom at all levels of existence – physical freedom through reduced tension and increased poise, emotional freedom through reduced anxiety and egocentricity and greater trust in the life flow, and mental and spiritual freedom through greater openness to being and broad relaxed attitudes.

It is surprising how much can be achieved by having in mind frequently throughout each day the conscious aim of letting go, of opening up, of being more relaxed and poised physically and mentally – once one has the knowledge and techniques to back up the aim.

## HUMOUR IS RELAXING

Lapses from poise in thought and behaviour should be mocked in good humour and their lessons noted. A touch of humour in relation to oneself, other people (the most frequent cause of tension) and the world in general is a relaxing touch.

The humourlessness of most religions is a drawback. Taoism and Zen are exceptions, being full of healthy belly-laughter – most of all at the Great Cosmic Joke.

Visitors calling at the home of Sigmund Freud were not offered a drink – but they were told a Jewish joke. Freud said the effect was the same – relaxing the visitor and putting him at ease. And jokes cost nothing at all!

When situations become too tense, too pompous, or too solemn, humour breaks it up and brings in laughter. Edward de Bono says that humour is a more significant process in the human mind than reason, because it enables us to switch from one way of looking at things to another. This is the way of creative thinking.

## RELAXED THINKING

Humour switches the patterns of thinking and stimulates new ideas; it is a tool of relaxed or Taoist thinking. Relaxed thinking is anti-rigid and anti-dogmatic, introduces discontinuity, humour, playfulness, feeling and new angles of approach to problems. Edward de Bono's lateral thinking is thinking of this type. Bringing together random and unlikely ideas is a fun tool for creativity at which children are often very good.

## EMPLOYMENT OF LEISURE

The poised person is likely to seek out the most deeply satisfying leisure activities, yet may be capable of moments of nonsense and lightheartedness. He or she takes pleasure in becoming absorbed in forms of creativity, which may take many forms. It would be pointless to attempt to specify activities, there are so many, and they are so much influenced by educational and cultural background, introversion and extraversion, and so on.

It is worth noting that when the whole person is committed to any activity it is satisfying and energy is available.

## FEELING FOR NATURE

A special feeling for Nature is a natural development of poised living and is expressed through contemplation: stop, look and listen. There will be special appreciation of the significance of the elements – of earth, water, air and fire. This feeling for Nature could be described as Taoist.

## DIRECT EXPERIENCE

The enjoyment of the significance of Nature comes from the life of sensation, from direct perception and direct experience. The distinction between the verbal, reflective level of experience and the non-verbal, bare attention experience should be clearly understood. Our verbal, conceptual picture of the world should not be imposed on the sensory experience of living, otherwise life becomes boring and trivial. Give bare and total attention to drinking a cup of tea and the simple act becomes meaningful. The evolutionary development of the cortical processes should not be allowed to rob life of its concrete reality and delight. Feeling rain on your forehead is important. So is gazing at the sea, eating an apple, and drinking a glass of wine.

Direct awareness of the constant flux of feelings and sensations may only be denied at the cost of health, loss of the sense of reality, and alienation from Nature that has produced us as a tree brings forth leaves. We are part of the cosmic dance whether we wish to or not. There is no opting out short of suicide.

Direct perception is the flint spark of mystical enlightenment, for which a library of verbal thinking is no substitute. This is strongly stated in Zen. 'Zen denies nothing,' wrote R. H. Blyth, 'has nothing negative in it, but it says, "Beware of Abstractions!"' When Fu-ketsu was asked by a monk how to transcend the relative world of both speaking and staying silent, the reply came immediately:

> I always think of Ko-Nan in March;
> Partridges chirp among the scented blossoms.

## SUBTLE INFLUENCES

Practice in detecting subtle tension in muscles should be extended to detecting all those things both great and small that cause psychic tension.

Pianist Sviatoslav Richter finds that blues and greys dominant in a concert-hall decor puts him in his most communicative mood. We are all artists – of living – and should become sensitive to the influence of colour in our lives, which is just one of many influences on tension and relaxation. The more we are aware of them, the more creative we can be in living.

## THE SERENITY PLATEAU

This book has been concerned with practical techniques that influence feelings, muscular and mental tone and states of consciousness. You should find that peace of mind can be attained and maintained, as though gliding through air, regardless of the normal vicissitudes of life.

Attitudes – underpinned by psychophysical training – make serenity possible. A poised, relaxed, open attitude makes a world of difference to the experience of living. André Maurois explained the importance of inner stance very well when he wrote: 'It is not events and the things one sees and enjoys that produced happiness, but a state of mind, which can endow events with its own quality, and we must hope for a duration of this state rather than the recurrence of pleasurable events.'

You can do more than hope for the state to arise and to persist – you can cultivate it and learn how to keep it flowing on. To know the purest happiness of the gliding kind, which is serenity, relaxation of the profoundest kind is essential. You need to let go from the anxiety and the dis-ease that prevents awareness (remembrance) of *being*.

## SELF-ACTUALIZATION: A PSYCHOLOGY OF BEING

The person living a relaxed, poised life is likely to manifest certain characteristics of personality and behaviour which would need a whole book to describe adequately. Some of these characteristics have already been mentioned – such as a special feeling for nature and a sense of humour. Others are: tolerance; broad non-rigid, non-fanatical beliefs; loving for its own sake; appreciating beauty, whether in nature or created by artist, poet or composer; appreciating things for their own sakes rather than for what the ego can get out of them; concern with being rather than with becoming, and with being rather than with having – a characteristic that the world badly needs today and well discussed by Erich Fromm in *To Have or To Be*; not being obsessed with material possessions, yet not dropping out of society; not being pushed or pulled, not impelled, freedom from conditioning; non-interference, letting be, yet also being responsible and caring (by watching and listening carefully, mindfulness of other people's feelings and needs).

The characteristics that I would expect to find in people who become experts in relaxation and poise carried through into the personality structure and the texture of living experience are by and large those described by Abraham H. Maslow (who died 1970) as belonging to men, women and children manifestly in process of actualizing their growth potential. Maslow called the process *self-actualization*.

In 1939 Kurt Goldstein had used the term self-actualization to explain the way brain-injured soldiers reorganized their capacities after injury. Other names for the tendency towards psychological health in human beings, more or less synonymous with self-actualization, are growth, self-realization, self-development, individuation and autonomy. These are terms used by psychologists of humanistic, third force psychology – the other two forces are Freudianism and behaviourism.

Maslow was a pioneer of the new force in psychology, which was firmly established by the late 1960s, with a large literature. Hitherto psychology had mostly been a study of mental ill-health; humanistic psychology looks mainly at psychological health. Maslow's book *Toward a Psychology of Being* (1962) has had a huge sale for a book of this type. In his preface to the second edition, Maslow said that

Third Psychology is now one facet of a general *Weltanschauung*, a new philosophy of life, a new conception of man, the beginning of a new century of work. . . . It helps to generate a way of life, not only for the person himself within his own private psyche, but also for the same person as a social being, a member of society.

The 'way of life' Maslow described is by and large that which I have in mind as 'poised living'. If I say that it is an updating of the old Chinese philosophical Taoism, in the light of modern psychological investigation, I do not believe I am forcing matters – Maslow himself frequently used the word Taoist to describe the characteristics of self-actualizing people.

These characteristics of healthy people tend to appear when the basic needs for safety, belongingness, love, respect and self-esteem have been gratified. These psychologically healthy people have increased spontaneity, detachment, autonomy, life-affirmation, acceptance of themselves, other people and nature, creativity, sense of reality, capacity to love and ego-transcendence. They tend to have more peak experiences.

Self-actualizing people do not lack ego strength, but they can be self-forgetful in work, play and interpersonal relations – 'absorption in perceiving, in doing, in enjoying, in creating can be very complete, very integrated and very pure'. They may not be socially withdrawing, but they know how to get enrichment from periods of solitude. To switch momentarily to the psychology of Karen Horney, they are not compelled either to move away from people or to move towards or against them. They are not compelled in any direction, being resistant to enculturation and not so much at the mercy of conditioning as other people. They can be unconventional when they want to be, but most of the time fit easily into the society in which they live.

They have a great capacity for love, though appear to need only a little of it in return. And now we come to the closeness of growth-motivated people 'to the realm of Being . . . this area dimly seen but nevertheless having undoubted basis in reality.' Maslow contrasts D-love (Deficiency love) with B-love (Being love). The former is like a hole which has to be filled, and when not filled leads to disease. When deficiency needs are met, the higher being qualities tend to be actualized. Being love is unselfish because it is not driven by a deficiency need; it is non-possessive, enjoyed for its own sake, and never sated. It has the qualities of an aesthetic or mystical peak experience.

## PEAK EXPERIENCES

There are some self-actualizing people who do not have peak experiences, or at least not peak experiences of marked intensity. Maslow mentioned Eleanor Roosevelt in this connection.

But in most healthy self-actualizing people peak experiences are both more frequent and more important. They cherish these flarings of delight and meaningfulness as touchstones of held values that make life worth living.

Maslow said that people in peak experiences 'for the time become self-actualizers'. These moments of delight, happiness, ecstasy and ego-transcendence are healthy. They are often connected with contemplation of nature, listening to music, looking at paintings, reading poetry, religious feeling, sexual love, parental love and the oceanic feeling of being at one with the universe or universal Being. The experience of Zen 'awakening' (satori or kensho), has all the characteristics of being an extremely powerful peak experience.

The regular practice of deep relaxation and of meditation, and the cultivation of poised living, predisposes people towards having more peak experiences and towards self-actualizing.

The peak experience is marked by what Maslow calls B-cognition (cognition of Being). There is total attention: what is seen is seen as though it is the whole of Being. People are seen as unique individuals. One factor links up with our earlier discussion of habituation. Repeated B-cognizing makes perception richer; things of beauty are enjoyed more and more; people are loved more and more. In contrast, when perception is anxiety-based or deficiency-determined, the first viewing satisfies the need. Self-actualizers do and enjoy things for their own sake. The peak experience is self-validating: it is an end experience and not means to an end. It justifies living.

In the peak experience, whether religious, philosophical, aesthetic, creative or sensory delight, there is a sense of wonder, of receiving, of 'choiceless awareness', of desirelessness, of letting go and of opening up. While ordinary cognition is fatiguing, Being-cognition is effortless and refreshing.

## BEING VALUES

These values of the self-actualizer are those again that I would associate with persons advanced in poised living: wholeness, aliveness, simplicity, truth, beauty, goodness, effortlessness, simplicity and self-sufficiency. These values in experience fuse with each other.

In the peak experience opposites are resolved – the *yin* and the *yang*, female and male, darkness and light, and so on. This is Taoist experience.

In peak experiences there is a sense of being outside time and space. It is an experience of oneness, flow and timelessness. This is true of any strong experience of direct perception when the verbalized concept of the object is not confused with the reality of the object. It is when we start thinking and verbalizing that we introduce time and space, birth and death, beginning and end. The verbal level of abstracting has its place, but most of us could do with spending more time on the non-verbal level. The great questions about the meaning of Life and so on admit of no answers on their own verbal level. But on the direct non-verbal level, life becomes, in the words of the Dutch philosopher van der Leuw, not a problem to be solved but a mystery to be enjoyed.

## PLATEAU LIVING

As well as writing about peak experiences, Maslow wrote about 'plateau living' and this is relevant to any concept of poised living. In time, and for many people it can be a surprisingly short time, if you follow the practical programme of this book, you may raise your total life experience to a level of well-being that at one time might have been that of a minor peak. At times you may still experience anxiety, fear, anger, hatred, envy and other negative and potentially dangerous emotions, but they become rarer and their impact is softened. If you look at such emotions with bare attention they fade away soon. Your ups no longer contrast as much with your downs, and you live with almost permanent equanimity.

Maslow did not believe that the peak experience could be produced at will, but only attained indirectly – for example, through devotion to some life interest. There are two kinds of peak experience – those that are accompanied by a sense of thrilling excitement (scoring a winning goal, seeing it scored, Nietzsche on the mountain in a storm) and those that are profoundly relaxing, melting, peaceful. There is also the plateau experience which is not brief and soaring like the peak experience, but is of Schubertian 'heavenly length' and is serene, even and purely enjoyed. Maslow gives the example of a mother quietly watching her baby playing or an elderly man contemplating the sea and knowing that its surf will go on for ever unlike his own life.

Maslow wrote that unlike the peak experience, plateau experience often can be evoked at will, after patient cultivation and learning.

The practice of bare attention will prove invaluable in cultivating the plateau experience. Many people learn to evoke the experience by listening to selected music or by reading certain poetry. Contemplation of Nature is probably the most universal means of eliciting the plateau experience of elevated serenity.

The Japanese tea ceremony is a formal exercise in the plateau experience, and plateau experiences await the person who cultivates sensitivity to the delights of Zen art and poetry.

Taoist, Ch'an and Zen art balances form with emptiness in a way that makes us aware of infinity and silences the yapping of our egos. Forms emerge (are born) out of emptiness. The sense of emptiness, of infinite space, is a major factor in the feeling of relaxation we get from this art. The black and white of ink painting or the restrained use of watercolour imparts a mood of directness and simplicity. There is also often carefreeness, purposelessness and humour. Tramps and rascals appear in Zen art. Alan Watts wrote in *The Way of Zen* that 'the aimless life is the constant theme of Zen art of every kind, expressing the artist's own inner state of going nowhere in a timeless moment.'

The state of 'no mind' and of purposelessness is expressed in Ch'an and Zen art, as is the Taoist spirit of *wu-wei* – in this case 'painting by not painting'.

The Japanese have words that are untranslatable to describe subtleties of response to the purposeless moments of life. There are the four basic moods collectively called *furyu*, for which only approximate interpretations are possible. *Sabi* is a mood of solitude, as evoked when alone and watching the silent fall of snow; *wabi* is a mood of gentle sadness that comes from seeing ordinary things in their 'suchness'; *aware* is a kind of nostalgia for things once loved that have passed away; and *yugen* is the sense of strangeness and mystery one gets on seeing mist over the sea or hills at dusk.

To explore the nuances of the Zen response to the fluctuating moods of nature is to become aware of one's own mood-blindness and mood-deafness. But this sensitivity, like the plateau experience itself, may be cultivated.

The qualities found in Zen art may be found also in Zen poetry. The short, seventeen-syllable haiku catches the instantaneous essence of the living moment as accurately and as meaningfully as Henri Cartier-Bresson catches the 'decisive moment' with his miniature camera. The live moment in its 'suchness' is the theme of both Zen art and Zen poetry. One relaxes, stays still, opens up and receives their impact directly, responding immediately. Alan Watts pointed out how silence plays the role in haiku that empty space does in Zen art.

Haiku are only sometimes obviously poetic. They often depict ordinary things, yet somehow make them meaningful.

How does one explain the effect of Buson's

> Fallen leaves!
> When the wind blows from the west
> They gather in the east.

The poet relies on the reader's feeling for nature and for autumn. Perhaps, too, a feeling for the natural order, acceptance of which represents the true freedom – the kind of feeling which gave D. T. Suzuki his greatest depth of realization on thinking of the Zen phrase 'the elbow does not bend outwards'.

The Zen poet supplies the bare facts resulting from bare attention, and we supply the rest through our response. Ernest Hemingway achieved similar effects by similar means in his prose. Read, for example, the ending of *A Farewell to Arms*, starting with the words: 'I went into the room and stayed with Catherine until she died. . . .' Hemingway's prose makes us share the bare attention of the narrator of the novel. Of course the 'art that conceals art' lies in the choice of words and their arranging.

Professor R. H. Blyth, an authority on the history of haiku, was able to write a bulky work on *Zen in English Literature and Oriental Classics*, though he did not include Hemingway.

Maslow was aware that some mystics, following illumination through peak experiences, are able to live at the high plateau level of unitive consciousness. The literature of mysticism gives accounts of this. In Zen and other Eastern mystical disciplines, enlightenment is not considered of real worth until it has illuminated everyday consciousness with its quality and insight.

The stages in Zen training are represented by a famous set of pictures – The Ten Oxherding Pictures – which go back to Chinese sources. The ox is the enlightenment experience of seeing into one's true nature. The various stages depicted of searching for the ox, finding its footprints, catching a glimpse of the ox, catching the ox, taming it, and so on, culminate in the tenth picture in which the man is barefoot and barechested, smiling broadly, mixing with the ordinary people in the market place. He carries a gourd of liquor for sharing with others. For him, the mountains are mountains again and the rivers are rivers. It is interesting to contrast the relaxed carefree spirit of the Zen enlightened man with the piety of some of the saints of other spiritual traditions.

## A PHILOSOPHY OF RELAXATION

Most of the elements in Zen which interest us in connection with poised living were the contributions of Taoism to Ch'an Buddhism. When Buddhism was taken from India to China, it acquired a direct and concrete nature through contact with the practical, realistic mind of the Chinese. This was Ch'an

Buddhism, which in Japan was called Zen Buddhism. Ch'an and Zen both mean 'meditation', and derive from the Sanskrit *dhyana*.

In Abraham H. Maslow's collection of papers published as *The Farther Reaches of Human Nature*, Taoism is mentioned on thirty-three pages and Zen on seven pages. The characteristics and values of self-actualizers are very Taoist. He called for scientists and therapists to acquire a more Taoist attitude – non-intruding, non-controlling, non-judging, listening attentively to what nature and people have to say. Patients should be shown how to help themselves. He contrasted classical scientific objectivity with Taoist objectivity which he called 'love knowledge'.

Maslow's belief in the self-validating truth and healthiness of Being-values led him to propose reversing the usual procedure of judging attitudes and values by the authority of a religion. Instead, he suggested, try judging the worth of a religion from how far it embodies Being-values. 'B-values are definers of "true" or functional, usable, helpful religion,' Maslow wrote. 'This criterion is probably best satisfied now by a combination of Zen and Tao[ism] and Humanism.'

The religion Taoism would come poorly out of Maslow's test – but philosophical Taoism would get top marks. When Maslow used the epithet 'Taoist' so many times, it was the philosophical Taoism of Lao Tzu, Chuang Tzu, and Lieh Tzu that he had in mind. Their philosophy is a philosophy of relaxation and their books are inspirations to people aspiring to live in a poised way. The Taoist religion brought in alchemy, magic, searching for the elixir of immortality, longevity exercises, and other things in which the philosophical Taoists were either disinterested or of which they disapproved. Hereafter, any mention I make of Taoism will refer to philosophical Taoism.

Its most famous work is the *Tao Te Ching* (pronounced *dow* (as in dowager), *dir* (as in dirty), and *jing* (as in jingo). It is attributed to Lao Tzu, an older contemporary of Confucius, though some modern scholars dispute this, saying it is a much later collection of Taoist sayings. The work has a unity of style and thought that points to its having been written by one person.

The philosophical Taoists were against prime causes of anxiety and tension in people today just as in the Chinese of their own times: the craving for power, material goods, wealth, success, praise, publicity and violence toward oneself and others. They were against clinging to fixed opinions, self-assertion and professed morality. For some reason a great many people think that if you take away these things there is nothing left, man becomes an empty shell. The Taoists said that the best things in life are left: the world of nature, art in which the artist is a channel for expressing the Tao, all the pleasures of the physical life and of sensation, companionship and love. Above all, they recommended the life of contemplation and of flowing with the Tao.

The *Tao* is usually translated as 'Way', though the word is often used in Taoist literature in ways for which 'Nature' would be a proper equivalent. To live according to the Tao therefore is to live in harmony with Nature and with the natural order. It is the way of going along with the life flow, of not-forcing, of openness to being. Lao Tzu's favourite image for the Tao was of water, which accommodates itself to wherever it happens to be and does not despise the low ground. In the *Tao Te Ching* (chapter 8) we find:

> The greatest virtue is like water; it is good to all things.
> It attains the most inaccessible places without strife.
> Therefore it is like Tao.
> It has the virtue of adapting itself to its place.
> It is virtuous like the heart by being deep.
> It is virtuous like speech by being faithful.
> It is virtuous like government in regulating.
> It is virtuous like a servant in its ability.
> It is virtuous like action by being in season.
> And because it does not strive it has no enemies.
>
> (tr. W. G. Old)

Chuang Tzu tells of an old man swimming below a cataract and coming out unharmed. Asked how he did it, the old man says:

I have no way of doing this. There was my original condition to begin with; then habit growing into nature; and lastly acquiescence in destiny. Plunging in with the whirl, I came out with the swirl. I accommodate myself to the water, not the water to me. And so I am able to deal with it after this fashion. . . . I was born upon dry land . . . and accommodated myself to dry land. That was my original condition. Growing up on the water, I accommodated myself to the water. That was what I meant by nature. And doing as I did without being conscious of any effort so to do, that was what I meant by destiny.

(tr. H. A. Giles)

The message of Lao Tzu, Chuang Tzu, and Lieh Tzu is the same: all things are united in the Tao, relax in harmony with the universe.

The books of Chuang Tzu and Lieh Tzu, written probably in the fifth and fourth centuries BC, may be looked on as commentaries on the *Tao Te Ching*, which has been translated more frequently than any other work except the Bible. The archaic Chinese from which it is translated allows of many interpretations, which is part of its fascination. If you love the *Tao Te Ching*, as many people do and have done over the years, you will not tire of reading different translations. The work casts its spell in all of them, inspires people to let go to the watercourse way of nature. This book of eighty-one short chapters and just over 5000 words (or characters) has been a major influence on Chinese thought and culture for about 2500 years, and through Ch'an Buddhism on Japanese culture.

There are some interesting parallels between the *Tao Te Ching* and the New Testament. Holmes Welch in *The Parting of the Way* lists fifteen parallels.

The Taoist principle of *wu-wei* (pronounced woo-way), or 'non-action' does not mean that one should as far as possible do nothing. It means not forcing, not going against the grain (*li*) or the natural flow. It means working with the life force – to work against the natural order brings trouble, as man has found in ecological matters. Forcing against the current produces ill-health and unhappiness. Wu-wei is the life style of the follower of the Tao. It is stooping to conquer, as the springy willow may be said to do under a load of snow, so that the snow slips off. The pine branch, in contrast, is rigid, does not yield and breaks under the weight of the snow.

### *Tao Te Ching*, 76:

Man at his birth is supple and tender, but in death he is rigid and strong.

It is the same with everything.

Trees and plants in their early growth are pliant and soft, but at the end they are withered and tough.

Thus rigidity and strength are concomitants of death, but softness and gentleness are companions of life.

(tr. W. G. Old)

The skilled boxer rolls with the punch, the skilled yachtsman trims his sails to the wind. In judo yielding leads to the overthrow of one's opponent, who is the victim of his own momentum. Though effort may be applied, it is done at the right time. Wu-wei is the skilful use of one's energies, effort wedded to effective timing. This timing is the secret of the craftsman's skills as well as those of the dancer or the sportsman. Taoist and Zen literature gives many examples of how the right mental attitude combines with physical skills in the creativity of the carpenter, the butcher, the wheelwright, and so on.

There is a cognitive factor: the expert in wu-wei uses his intelligence to see the easiest and at the same time the most effective ways to do things, whether it be sawing wood or governing a nation. Lao Tzu's advice to rulers was to govern as one cooked small fish – lightly. He also saw the wisdom of small units for good government – the 'small is beautiful' concept.

The *Tao Te Ching* may be interpreted at several different levels. It is a treatise on mystical wisdom, on governing, on ecology; a book of natural philosophy; and a manual of poised living, the oldest and most inspiring. The basic technique that Lao Tzu gave was that given at physical and psychological levels in this book – *letting go*. By letting go, whether you belong to the East or to the West, you gain real relaxation and peace of mind.

> The student learns by daily increment,
> The Way is gained by daily loss,
> Loss upon loss until
> At last comes rest.

Following the Tao is the gentle art of poised living, by which ordinary living is effortless flow and constant celebration. Chuang Tzu wrote of this letting go from psychophysical tension, this emptying of the self:

To him who does not dwell in himself, the forms of things show themselves as they are. His movement is like that of water; his stillness is like that of a mirror; his response is like that of the echo. His rarefied condition makes him seem to be disappearing altogether; he is still as a clear lake, harmonious in his association with others. . . .

# Bibliography

Assagioli, Roberto, *Psychosynthesis*, Viking Press, New York, 1971.

Barker, Sarah, *The Alexander Technique: The Revolutionary Way to Use your Body for Total Energy*, Bantam Books, New York, 1978.

Barlow, Wilfrid, *The Alexander Principle*, Gollancz, London, 1973.

Benson, Herbert, M.D. *The Relaxation Response*. William Morrow, New York, 1976.

Blythe, Peter, *Self-hypnosis: Its Potential and Practice*, Arthur Barker, London, 1976.

Blyth, R. H., *Zen and Zen Classics*, vol.1, Hokuseiso Press, Japan, 1960.

Blyth, R. H., *Zen in English Literature and Oriental Classics*, E. P. Dutton, New York, 1973.

Bogert, L. Jean, *Nutrition and Physical Fitness*.

Brown, Barbara B., *New Mind, New Body*, Harper & Row, New York, 1974; Hodder & Stoughton, London, 1977.

Brown, Barbara B., *Stress and the Art of Biofeedback*, Harper & Row, New York, 1977.

Bucke, Richard Maurice, *Cosmic Consciousness: A Study in the Evolution of the Human Mind*, University Books, New York, 1961; Olympia Press, 1972.

Byles, Marie Beuzeville, *Stand Straight Without Strain: The Original Exercises of F. Matthias Alexander*, Fowler, Romford, Essex, 1978.

Cade, C. Maxwell, and Coxhead, Nona, *The Awakened Mind: Biofeedback and the Development of Higher States of Awareness*, Wildwood House, London, 1979.

De Bono, Edward, *Lateral Thinking*, Cape, London, 1967.

De Bono, Edward, *PO: Beyond Yes and No*, Simon & Schuster, New York, 1972.

Feng, Gia Fu, and English, Jane, *Tao Te Ching*, Alfred A. Knopf, New York, 1972; Wildwood House, London, 1973.

Fenton, Jack Vinten, *Choice of Habit: Poise, Free Movement, and the Practical Use of the Body*, Macdonald & Evans, London, 1973.

Fromm, Erich. *To Have and to Be*, Harper and Row, New York, 1976; Jonathan Cape, London, 1978.

Fromm, Erich; Suzuki, D. T.; De Martino, Richard, *Zen Buddhism and Psychoanalysis*, Harper and Row, New York, 1960; Souvenir Press, London, 1974.

Giles, Herbert A. (tr.), *Chuang Tzu: Mystic, Moralist, and Social Reformer*, Kelly and Walsh, Shanghai, 1926.

Goleman, Daniel, *The Varieties of the Meditative Experience*, Rider, London, 1978.

Hartland, John, *Medical and Dental Hypnosis and Its Clinical Application*, Ballière, Tindall and Cassell, London, 1966.

Hewitt, James, *New Faces*, A. Thomas, Wellingborough, Northants, 1977.

Hewitt, James, *Teach Yourself Meditation*, Hodder Stoughton, London, 1978.

Hewitt, James, *Teach Yourself Yoga*, Hodder & Stoughton, London, 1979.

Hewitt, James, *Isometrics: The Short Cut to Fitness*, Thorsons, Wellingborough, Northants, 1980.

Jacobson, Edmund, MD, *Progressive Relaxation*, University of Chicago Press, 1929.

Jacobson, Edmund, MD, *You Must Relax*, McGraw-Hill, New York, 1962.

Kapleau, Philip, *The Three Pillars of Zen: Teaching, Practice, Enlightenment*, Beacon Press, Boston, 1967, Rider, London, 1980.

Kapleau, Philip, *Zen: Dawn in the West*, Rider, London, 1980.

Krishnamurti, J., *Commentaries on Living* (third series), Victor Gollancz, London, 1962.

Lao Tzu, *Tao Te Ching* (tr. W. G. Old), Rider, London, 1904.

Linssen, Robert, *Living Zen*, Grove Press, New York, 1960; Allen and Unwin, London, 1958.

Marcuse, F. L., *Hypnosis, Fact and Fiction*, Penguin Books, Harmondsworth, Middx, 1959.

Maslow, Abraham H., *Motivation and Personality*, Harper & Row, New York, 1954.

Maslow, Abraham H., *Toward a Psychology of Being*, D. Van Nostrand, New York, 1968.

Maslow, Abraham H., *The Farther Reaches of Human Nature*, Viking Press, New York, 1971.

Naranjo, Claudio, and Ornstein, Robert E., *On the Psychology of Meditation*, Allen & Unwin, London, 1972.

Nyanoponika Thera, *The Heart of Buddhist Meditation: A Handbook of Mental Training Based on the Buddha's Way of Mindfulness*, Rider, London, 1962.

Ornstein, Robert E., *The Psychology of Consciousness*, W. H. Freeman, San Francisco, 1972.

Ornstein, Robert E. (ed.), *The Nature of Human Consciousness*, W. H. Freeman, San Francisco, 1973.

Powys, John Cowper, *In Defence of Sensuality*, Victor Gollancz, London, 1930; Village Press, London, 1974.

Powys, John Cowper, *A Philosophy of Solitude*, Jonathan Cape, London, 1933; Village Press, London, 1974.

Powys, John Cowper, *The Art of Happiness*, Bodley Head, London, 1935; Village Press, London, 1975.

Rosa, Dr Karl Robert, *Autogenic Training*, Victor Gollancz, London, 1976.

Sekida, Katsuki, *Zen Training: Methods and Philosophy*, John Weatherhill, New York, 1975.

Sekiguchi, Shindai, *Zen: A Manual for Westerners*, Japan Publications, Tokyo.

Suzuki, Daisetz T., *An Introduction to Zen Buddhism*, Rider, London, 1949.

Suzuki, Daisetz T., *Zen and Japanese Culture*, Routledge & Kegan Paul, Romford, Essex, 1959.

Suzuki, Daisetz T., *The Field of Zen*, Harper & Row, New York, 1970.

Suzuki, D. T., Fromm, Erich, and Martino, Richard de, *Zen Buddhism and Psychoanalysis*, Harper & Row, New York, 1960; Souvenir Press, London, 1974.

Von Durckheim, Karlfried Graf, *Hara: The Vital Centre of Man*, Allen & Unwin, London, 1962.

Watts, Alan, *Beyond Theology*, Pantheon Books, New York, 1964; Hodder and Stoughton, London, 1964.

Watts, Alan, *The Way of Zen*, Pantheon Books, New York, 1957.

Watts, Alan, *Cloud-Hidden, Whereabouts Unknown*, Jonathan Cape, London, 1974.

Watts, Alan, *Tao: The Watercourse Way*, Jonathan Cape, London, 1976.

Weinberg, Harry L., *Levels of Knowing and Existence*, Harper & Row, New York, 1959.

Welch, Holmes, *The Parting of the Way*, Methuen, London, 1958; Beacon Press, Boston, 1966 (as *Taoism: The Parting of the Way*).

Wilson, Colin, *The Occult*, Hodder & Stoughton, London, 1971.

Wilson, Colin, *New Pathways in Psychology: Maslow and the Post-Freudian Revolution*, Victor Gollancz, London, 1972.

Wilson, Colin, *Mysteries*, Hodder & Stoughton, London, 1978.

# Index